Challenging Behaviour

Principles and Practices

Edited by

Dave Hewett

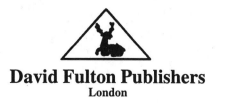

David Fulton Publishers
London

David Fulton Publishers Ltd
Ormond House, 26–27 Boswell Street, London WC1N 3JD

First published in Great Britain by David Fulton Publishers 1998

Note: The right of Dave Hewett to be identified as the editor of this work has been asserted by him in accordance with the Copyright, Designs and Patents Act 1988.

Copyright © David Fulton Publishers Ltd 1998

British Library Cataloguing in Publication Data
A catalogue record for this book is available from the British Library

ISBN 1–85346–451–1

Typeset by Textype Typesetters, Cambridge
Printed in Great Britain by BPC Books and Journals, Exeter

Contents

Acknowledgements

My thanks to John Carpenter, John Harris, David Hopkins, Penny Lacey, Liz Loftus, Simon Lowe, Liz Sharpe, Chris Sowter, Eva Timotheou, Rosemary Salter, Pamela Hawkins, the hard-working staff everywhere I have met during the last seven years, and especially Andy Arnett for talking, thinking, and 'The stages'. Ian Harris for manuscript reading and critical discussion; Stephen Swailes for the illustrations; Melanie Nind for all of the thinking together for so many years; Sarah Forde for her ability with computer software, the graphics, and generally being totally efficient and supportive.

Dedicated to the hard-working and harassed staff everywhere who like their jobs.

Introduction

Dave Hewett

This is a book about the everyday experiences of staff from various disciplines working with people with learning difficulties who have challenging behaviour. There are nine accounts about their work written by individuals or by groups of staff. The main purpose of the book is to provide the reader with descriptions of people attempting to achieve good practice, with which other practitioners could identify. I offer three commentary chapters which attempt to offer some practical theory and an overview to the work of the contributors. The emphasis is thus on the practicalities of what people do.

The contributors were invited to write for two reasons. Firstly they are 'ordinary' practitioners who are in their working situation day by day, doing their jobs, experiencing the ups and downs that are inevitable in what they are trying to achieve. Secondly, however, they are perhaps not ordinary in the extent to which they think about and reflect on their work, strive to improve their practice, work from and develop good principles, and thereby have something to offer by writing about what they do.

There is not a grand exposition of a single unifying psychological theory, though I have no objection to one and everything in this book is probably influenced by psychological thinking. The unifying theory, such as it is, shows staff working very hard at the ecology of their workplace, trying to create environments where challenging behaviour is less likely. Staff are shown to be working at coping with the challenging behaviours which occur, with sensible and humane practices, while doing everything in their power to help the person with the learning difficulty feel better, understand more and interact more positively. To achieve this it is necessary to think, talk, try things, think again, try again. It is also clear that the practitioners in this book have values and principles which are important to them and which guide their thinking and practice.

Only two of the people writing here have been previously published in the literature on working with people with severe learning difficulties. All of them have been encouraged to take on the rather daunting task of writing a chapter because I thought they had something worth sharing with other practitioners. For one contributor, Bernie Hunt, the task was a particularly massive one. She has a specific learning difficulty which means that the documentation of her day-to-day work is by no means impossible, but it is a laborious aspect of her job. For this reason, she and Peter Brooks 'wrote' their chapter in tape-recorded sessions with myself. I think that the interview format which resulted contributes to the diversity of writing styles present in the book.

The contributors have frequently drafted sections separately to make up their story. Where this occurs the name of the person writing is given in the title to each section, or ahead of several sections which have been penned by the same person.

Terminology

Geraint Ephraim (Chapter 12) offers astute observations on the use of the term 'challenging behaviour' and presents some alternative ways of thinking about them as 'exotic communications'. In many senses, I too have a preference for thinking about people's behaviours in terms of the thoughts and feelings which generate them. However, 'challenging behaviour' is the popular, universal term of the moment and this is the one used throughout the book and appearing in its title.

The contributors to the book are members of a range of professional disciplines and various words or phrases thus appear to describe the people with learning difficulties for whom they work: 'client', 'service-user', 'pupil', 'student'. In recent years I have become more accustomed to using the phrase 'service-user' as the least value-laden phrase which will describe all of the people for whom services make provision. Therefore I use the term generically in my contributions, implying a person in a school, day centre, residential establishment or college, though I use some of the other terms where appropriate.

The chapters and their contributors

Chapter 1 is a summary of unifying themes found in the contributions. I offer in addition some frameworks for meeting the needs of people who can be challenging. This is resolved into a positive conceptualisation for such work: 'helping the person learn how to behave'.

Martin Bertulis is the Principal of Womaston House, a residential school under the auspices of MacIntyre Care. In Chapter 2, with other staff, Paul Norton, Paul Jones, Carol Cadwallader, Pam Grounds and Steve McGreevy, he writes of their 'positive approaches' to challenging behaviour with reference to experiences with one particular pupil.

In Chapter 3, Nicki Bond and Don O'Connor of Hertfordshire Social Services describe their experiences in a small residential unit dedicated to the needs of a person with severely challenging behaviours.

Bernard Emblem is the headteacher of Millwood School in Bury, Lancashire. In Chapter 4 (with Jill Leonard, Karen Dale, Joanne Redmond, and Ruth Bowes) he details the hurly-burly of a lively classroom which has some particularly active and interesting pupils as members. He seeks to examine and rationalise the relaxed and seemingly natural working processes of his dedicated staff.

In Chapter 5, I set out what is offered as useful principles for managing incidents of challenging behaviour. The emphasis here is on staff being prepared with helpful and positive attitudes, thinking processes and structures – guidelines for what staff can do when the 'chips are down'.

Chapter 6 contributes to the breadth of service provision encompassed in the chapters. Bernie Hunt and Peter Brookes are respectively a lecturer and a student support assistant working for Oaklands College of Further Education in Hertfordshire. Their classroom is set within a long-stay hospital and is dedicated to meeting the needs of people with the more severely challenging behaviours.

Tracey Culshaw and Karin Purvis (Chapter 7) chronicle their experiences concerned with working toward unified and mutual work with a residential social services team in Somerset. Tracey was at that time the unit manager and Karin a speech and language therapist.

Chapter 8 is about a classroom for one. Maggie Roberts, a teacher, and Ann Vine, a teaching assistant, with East Sussex Education Authority, accepted posts as staff working with one young man for whom it was felt necessary to make individual provision, due to the nature of his challenges.

In Chapter 9, I move from principles to 'Managing incidents of challenging behaviour – practices', which is concerned with thinking about strategies for difficult situations, and includes the use of voice, body language and positioning.

Lewis Janes in Chapter 10 accounts his tribulations at becoming team leader of a social services residential provision in Somerset. His story is concerned with developing team work and team understandings, particularly for learning to cope with the challenges presented by a resident with a diagnosis of autism and some extreme anxieties.

In Chapter 11, Rosemary Hawkins, a teacher with Buckinghamshire Education Authority, describes her increasingly focused work on the communication needs of a pupil who was extremely difficult to reach. She highlights the theme of the relationship between communication, ability to relate and challenging behaviour.

In his own words, Geraint Ephraim is supposedly a visiting 'expert' psychologist, and in Chapter 12, he offers a wry commentary on his role and working life. At the same time, he makes fundamental, if not profound, observations about the sources of challenging behaviours, measures which staff need to undertake to help those who are challenging, and the difficulties and hazards facing staff doing this work.

Chapter 1

Commentary: helping the person learn how to behave

Dave Hewett

Introduction

Firstly a confessional, to assist the reader further with understandings about my orientation to the contents and purpose of this book. I started working with people with learning difficulties as a teacher, more than 20 years ago. Circumstances and some of my own preferences caused me quickly to gravitate to working with people who had challenging and, frequently, severely challenging behaviours.

In my early years, I was fortunate to work with some lovely colleagues who taught me many useful things about doing this work. It would also be true to say, however, that attitudes and practices were in general somewhat different in the mid 1970s. My experience was that there was a more easygoing attitude to what staff were allowed to do in order to control people's behaviour and to try to make the behaviour go away. Shouting, being angry and the use of casual physical force were much more in evidence as part of the staff's technique. I was one of these staff. Being allowed, or even expected, to indulge in that behaviour style unfortunately chimed in with some existing tendencies in my personality to indulge occasionally in angry and aggressive behaviour.

However, I moved on and changed. Bitter, often painful, experience taught me that it was very difficult to change people and the way people behaved simply by dominating them and demanding that they behave differently. I commenced a happy and as yet incomplete process of addressing the personal factors which contributed to my own occasional challenging behaviour. Significantly I started working with a staff group who increasingly dedicated themselves to cool, technical appraisals of the people and the challenging behaviours they were presented with. They dedicated themselves also to the development of the warmest and most understanding set of practices they could devise. Most of them were younger or less experienced than me, but with them I learnt proper calmness, how to defuse situations, how not to get into situations you didn't have to be in, and how to be truly relaxed and positive. We were working with people who were likely to provide the more severe challenges and we loved our work. I hope the reader will be comforted, however, by my mentioning that whatever criticisms of 'poor' practices might be implied by some of the points in this book, I have probably indulged in those practices.

The following chapters all describe practice which reflects the preferences I have developed for what should be the basis of good work with people's challenging behaviour. The intention is to describe the experiences of staff who enjoy working with people who are difficult to be with, who feel that they are, at the very least, effective as practitioners, and to give a feel for what it is that they do. The emphasis is on the practical and the basic, and the thought and discussion which goes with those things. This emphasis is much influenced by John Harris' formulation of 'everyday good practice' (Harris and Hewett 1996).

'Everyday good practice' implies the necessity for staff to put a great deal of thought and energy into developing positive attitudes and acquiring good interpersonal skills for managing people'schallenging behaviour effectively. Hand-in-hand with everyday good practice should be attention to needs such as making the environment agreeable, having good programmes of work for matters such as communication and relationships, helping people progress, develop and move forward, as well as teamwork and documentation of their work. If these basics are properly addressed, challenging behaviours can feel less challenging and most people will be less challenging.

Working with people's difficult feelings and the behaviour generated by them can seem like a complex affair, but it can be reduced to two straightforward aims:

- cope with the way that the person behaves at present;
- help the person to make progress and change.

Coping may be the aim which is frequently not properly attended to for several reasons. Staff can feel under a great deal of pressure to 'cure' people of challenging behaviour, and as quickly as possible. This aspiration can lead to inadequate time and energy being spent on developing good coping procedures. Some very human frailties can get in the way also. When a person'sbehaviour is particularly challenging, it can be easy to become so fixed on changing the person as a priority, that one forgets to put effort into coping. Additionally, a feeling of resentment that the person just should not be behaving like this, can also be a barrier to giving coping procedures the time and effort they deserve.

Most people do not change their lifestyle and behaviour easily and quickly, so it is good practice to make the priority the ability to cope well with the reality of how they presently behave. Staff groups who do this are then in a much better position to operate the second aim – to do good, effective work with the person on changing and moving forward with their abilities and understandings. The contributors show these two elements as essential strands in their work – a fundamental orientation to viewing their work in as simple and straightforward fashion as possible.

Themes present in the work of the contributors to this book

As well as those aims outlined above, other clear themes regularly recur in the stories of practice in this book. The contributors were selected partly because of the diversity of their working situations and the people with whom they work, yet the similarity of so much they describe about their work is a striking feature. Some of the more prominent themes are listed in Figure 1.1. These comprise what may be seen as a 'practical audit' of pointers to achieving good practice and each is discussed here in turn.

Acceptance that challenging behaviour occurs – it is normal

This is the most realistic attitude for staff working with people with learning difficulties to maintain. It can be difficult, especially if staff have 'curing' the person quickly as an absolute priority. Tracey Culshaw (Chapter 7) illustrates this. She worked hard with her staff to foster this viewpoint, she wanted it to be a central aspect of staff attitudes and practice. The possession of this attitude contributes to teams and individual members of staff developing practices whose starting point is compassion and understanding. It is one of the foundations of the

---

- acceptance that challenging behaviour occurs – it is normal

- there is a focus on much more than the negative behaviour – there is a dedication to improving the lifestyles and therefore the behaviour of the people with whom they work

- a quest for understanding: viewing challenging behaviour as a manifestation of complex inner state interacting with what is happening around the person

- emphasis on developing communication and relationship abilities

- emphasis on coping – positive, pragmatic incident management practices

- a sense of 'asylum' being available in their provision

- attending to all of the basic details of their practices

- collaboration, reflection and documentation

- teamwork and team practices

- constant thought on balancing service-users' rights with staff duty of care

- interest and enjoyment

Figure 1.1 Themes present in the work of the contributors

staff's ability to remain calm in difficult circumstances and to deal effectively with their own feelings of anger and frustration. It is not in contradiction of the next item below; effective staff maintain both of these viewpoints simultaneously.

There is a focus on much more than the negative behaviour – there is a dedication to improving the lifestyles, and therefore the behaviour, of the people with whom they work

The writers here all show the lack of surprise, indignation or resentment at the styles of behaviour they are presented with, which is implicit in the acceptance stressed above. This acceptance does not impede their desire or drive to help each person to find more profitable and rewarding ways of interacting with the people around them. They are able to have an approach which does much more than negatively focus on eradicating the challenging behaviour. They pay attention to many aspects of the person's lifestyle, attempting to enrich it and diversify it, particularly in respect of social understandings and social interaction. There is a fundamental belief that doing this is more effective than simply focusing on eradicating the unwanted behaviour.

A quest for understanding: viewing challenging behaviour as a manifestation of complex inner state interacting with what is happening around the person.

All contributors describe their thoughts on what contributes to the behaviour of the person they are working with. None of them view it as a straightforward issue – there is no great search for the single 'cause' of the person's behaviour and a correspondingly 'quick fix'. They are all sensitive to the 'triggers' of challenging incidents, and there are good examples of approaches to dealing with triggers – by removing them where possible, managing the effects of them where it is not. However, they do not confuse the trigger with the cause of the person's behaviour. The practitioners writing here recognise the degree to which various factors come together to 'cause' the way that a person behaves and to create possible triggers. Nicki Bond and Don O'Connor (Chapter 3) offer a stark list of some of the factors they judge to be present in Andrew's behaviour. Helping the person to move forward and develop more positive interactions with the world may sometimes be a seemingly complex and painstaking affair of working on the contributory factors inside the person and paying attention to and changing wherever possible, the contributing factors outside the person.

This approach to viewing the causes of the person's behaviour is illustrated in Figure 1.2 and 1.3. The lists are not exhaustive, but they outline some of the more usual factors which are likely to contribute to the challenging behaviour of people with learning difficulties in our services. (Actually, the lists are useful for all of us in thinking about our own occasional challenging behaviours.) They give a

4

Personal factors

Genetics, e.g.
- genetic conditions which are thought to influence behaviour directly

Constitutional or physiological, e.g.
- hormonal state
- hunger/food/thirst
- allergies
- brain damage
- drug regimes
- illness
- epilepsy
- mental health problems
- mobility/physical abilities
- physical pain

Relationships
- difficulty experiencing understandable relationships
- understandable relationships not available

Personality and character, e.g.
- limited emotional development – emotions still 'raw'
- extremes of extroversion or introversion
- neuroticism
- impulsiveness
- limited knowledge about enjoying life, having fun, finding each passing moment pleasurable
- changeable moods
- arousal pattern, e.g. high arousal 'normal' state
- coping styles (ability to cope with own emotions)
- unstable early upbringing experiences

Sense of self, e.g.
- self-esteem – unable to see self as valuable – as 'good to be with'
- self-view, e.g. 'this is how I am' – seeing self as a difficult or violent person
- degree of self-knowledge/insight
- feelings of powerlessness

Damage
- e.g. sexual or physical, or emotional/psychological abuse
- first-hand experience of e.g. violence
- history of challenging behaviour – routine part of lifestyle

Difficulty with communication, e.g.
- not able to use nor understand language
- difficulty with verbal expression and understanding
- difficulty with understanding others, e.g. perceptual problems

Basic needs and abilities, e.g.
- still not socialised into the way of behaving shared by other people due to communication/relationship difficulties
- unfulfilled sexual needs
- still at early developmental stage
- still has basic security and social needs

Figure 1.2 Common personal factors underlying the production of challenging behaviour

Environmental factors

Quality of physical environment, e.g.
- lighting
- acoustics
- noise levels
- space available
- humidity
- heating
- colours

Quality of the social environment, e.g.
- general social complexity – too many people too near
- environment not complex enough – unstimulating
- environment has challenging behaviour normally occurring
- staff interaction styles not sensitive to person's present abilities

Places in position of powerlessness, e.g.
- being extensively goal-blocked
- unreasonable punishment
- extensive use of punishment
- lack of access of decision making
- lack of access to choice over own actions
- staff stress on compliance and conformity
- staff reliance on confrontation and win/lose scenarios
- behaviour constantly scrutinised with freuent interventions from staff
- staff focus on behaviour more than feelings

Unpredictable occurrences, e.g.
- being startled/cornered
- lack of understanding about what is happening in the environment
- other people's outbursts

Other people's high expectations, e.g.
- 'good' behaviour always
- behave your chronological age always
- staff set unachievable objectives

All communication difficulties, e.g.
- lack of access to communications at own level of ability
- lack of access to communications with staff
- staff lack expertise in communication activities
- communication difficulties between staff – staff not 'getting their act together', working consistently with shared understandings

Figure 1.3 Common environmental factors underlying the production of challnging behaviour

framework for thinking about the aim of helping the person with challenging behaviour to progress and change. They should assist with the development of the sort of work that the contributors carried out on starting to get the world right, working on communication, relationship and well-being, the elements of the environment which interact with personal factors. Simply sitting together and using the lists to do a brain-storm with a service-user as the subject, can be a significant experience for staff teams. The written results can bring home the reality that a great many serious influences are contributing to the behaviour of the person and that it is understandable that she/he indulges in some behaviours which are difficult to deal with.

This conceptualisation underpins the approaches in the various chapters. The contributors are not seeking simply to make the behaviour go away and view that as the job done. They consider the likely factors affecting their service-users, put in place a range of initiatives which address these factors and work to have an environment which is as agreeable as possible. There is even the perception that the people writing here would not be content in their work if the challenging behaviours stopped, but the person with learning difficulties was still unhappy, distressed or isolated.

There is great concern for how people with challenging behaviour view themselves – the issues of self-esteem and self-view. Work on communication and relationship goes hand-in-hand with these issues and is likely to contribute mightily to a person's self-worth if she/he is having regular positive valuing experiences in interactions with others. This is an area which might require great thought and professionalism, however. It can be very difficult indeed to give, or even desire to give, positive human experiences to a person who is difficult to be with and generally displays negative or abusive behaviour towards others. There is no doubt that these positive experiences are necessary and likely to increase people's sense of feeling good about themselves, resulting in positive effects in their behaviour. It is only recently that discussion of issues of self-esteem have become more prominent in work with people with learning difficulties (see also Clements 1997, Stenfort Kroese 1997). Whilst the discussion here is short, I would hope that the reader none the less recognises its status as a major issue in the work of the contributors.

While working with a concept of factors may seem to be a complex undertaking, there is none the less also a strong sense that the staff writing here view it as a logical and highly practical way of working. They are also flexible, reviewing their conceptualisations of their service-user's state and modifying their action plans accordingly. No procedures become 'carved in stone', staff complacency can turn out to be a significant environmental factor in challenging behaviour occurring.

Emphasis on developing communication and relationship abilities

There is striking repetition of these issues in the accounts. Rosemary Hawkins' work (Chapter 11) with Ann is fully focused on these factors, in recognition that her behaviour is part of a lifestyle formed by her limited abilities to make contact with other people. Although Ann was 'full of life', little of it was concerned with relating to others. One of the major contributing forces to a person learning to have ordered behaviour is the effect and influence of other people's behaviour on them. If the person has limited ability to relate and communicate with others, she/he has correspondingly limited opportunity to be socialised into the ways of behaving shared by others. This recognition of a person's ability should have a fundamental effect, as it did for Rosemary Hawkins, on the extent to which people with very severe learning difficulties are expected to have self-control and be 'disciplined' by external forces. Realistically, they may have little ability to respond in this way. This does not mean that staff should not be doing what they can to control the person, but it does mean that such attempts to control should take into account the person's actual ability to have self-control and be set also within a more far-ranging application of effort on communication and relating.

Although Ann presents us with the most extreme example of this state of affairs, the issue applies equally to the work of contributors who may be caring for or teaching people with more developed abilities. They all recognise the absolutely fundamental nature of communication in human behaviour and that lack of social understanding results in so much difficulty. Karin Purvis (Chapter 7) illustrates this application even with people who have apparently extensive ability to speak and understand speech. In my work with the staff group I described earlier, we powerfully formed the view that even small improvements in communication ability could have correspondingly beneficial and welcome outcomes in terms of behaviour (see Nind and Hewett 1994). The message from the contributors here is simply, never have a behaviour programme – without also having a communication programme.

An emphasis on coping – positive, pragmatic incident management practices

Coping first and foremost is a major theme of the accounts. Coping well with the person's behaviour and all aspects of the working situation is attended to in detail. Some of the writers, notably Maggie Roberts (Chapter 8) and Nicki Bond and Don O'Conner (Chapter 3) may be considered fortunate to have working situations where appropriate time could be devoted to these considerations, without the compromises necessitated by the conflicting needs of more than one student or client. However, the work of Bernard Emblem's (Chapter 4) staff also illustrates the team pragmatically adjusting themselves to the reality of the behaviours they were presented with. This was partly influenced by whether the person actually has the ability to be 'controlled', but also by some seemingly natural serenity on the part of the staff. The result was some realistic and practical approaches to incidents, coping well with what takes place, while working hard at all other times to help the person progress.

There is also the reality that coping can take time. Lewis Janes and his staff (Chapter 10) worked through some long situations with Brenda. Their 'patience' was partly founded on a realistic appraisal of the consequences if they did not give the time necessary, and partly on an implicit understanding of Brenda's unavoidable and deep anxiety.

Bernie Hunt and Peter Brooks (Chapter 6) are articulate about the psychological basis of being able to cope. They are, so to speak, 'hard-bitten' campaigners in their experience of dealing with themselves, their own personal responses and those of other staff, to people's outrages. For them, coping with themselves is second-nature as the first step in coping with others and objectively carrying out all of the practicalities necessary.

Coping extends to pragmatic approaches to working with incidents of challenging behaviour. These practicalities are discussed in more detail in Chapter 9, but the contributors share strong, common themes in their approach to those circumstances. They share a preference to defusing situations rather than dominating them. They operate essential priorities in managing incidents: focus on what is taking place, manage the incident in an uncomplicated fashion, achieve an effective outcome. On the whole they resist attempting to do other things during incidents, recognising that mostly, this is not a good time for the person to conduct positive learning. Also, it is probably not the best time to do things aimed at not having another incident. Their efforts in these areas tend to be at all other times. However, they do value the positive cumulative affect that the service-user is likely to derive from being dealt with consistently at difficult moments by staff who are calm, ordered and understanding. They are also realistic about the time that challenging behaviour can take up.

Although I have described this orientation to managing the worst moments of behaviour as pragmatic, it is also influenced by the contributors' beliefs and values. The understanding derived from viewing the person's behaviour as a result of a multiplicity of factors, with the person not therefore held solely responsible for it, is one. The simple perception that the incident is a bad time for education since the person is, for understandable reasons, in a bad state, is another value-driven attitude – as well as being pragmatic. I think the writers are also concerned about their own self-view. They share what seems to be a deep desire to have practices which they themselves can approve of as human beings – doing the right thing in terms of ethics, human rights and their personal conception of the human condition.

A sense of 'asylum' being available in their provision and practices

Martin Bertulis (Chapter 2) specifically refers to this need. 'Asylum' is a somewhat old-fashioned word and it is full of negative connotations. However, Martin's plea is not just about the status of his establishment as a place well away from everyone else out in the countryside. He is making the point, which I think is endorsed by the work of the other contributors, that in our work there must be some sort of time and place for people to behave in a way which reflects what and who they are. This is not to be seen as a contradiction with aspiring to help them progress, it is a part of it.

For some, perhaps many people with learning difficulties, the pressure of matters such as ordinary living, age-appropriate behaviour and having good, ordered behaviour at all times can be very great. This is especially so if the gap between these expectations and the way they feel, and are therefore likely to behave, is very great. In a sense the pressure imposed by these expectations may become another environmental factor in their behaviour.

Any programme of activities and practices aimed at helping a person move forward and develop, must surely have as one of its premises tolerance, time and space for a person to behave the way they feel. Some people with challenging behaviours are so uncompromising with their lifestyle that this acceptance is forced on the staff working with them. Martin Bertulis, Bernie Hunt and Peter Brooks, the staff group of Flat 7 (Chapter 3), work in situations at this end of the spectrum. However, many other people who challenge only occasionally can be mostly compliant in a way that can hide their emotional needs and true feelings. There may be a need for services to have, therefore, a far greater acceptance of their occasional outbursts rather than less tolerance, because their ability to behave well at other times is so great.

Attending to all of the basic details of their practices

The concept of everyday good practice mentioned earlier is in evidence in the accounts here, together with an, at times, remorseless attention to the detail of the writers' working environments. Again, although these practitioners are operating a positive yet complex view of behaviour and its contributory factors, the sheer practicality of how they attend to their working situation is a powerful message. Nicki Bond and Don O'Connor (Chapter 3) write in almost amused revelation of their growing discovery of the need to attend to the minute routines which observed Andrew's sense of well-being. Rosemary Hawkins (Chapter 11) chronicles the detail of the thinking and planning that went into the development of their approach with Ann. At the same time a great deal of flexibility was needed to meet the new contingencies created by each new initiative.

Working in this way – attending to detail, being flexible, being prepared constantly to revamp what is done – can be one of the more difficult aspects of the work for staff working under pressure. The ability to do it will also be fundamentally affected by teamworking processes, particularly the ability of people to talk to each other. It is difficult to have effective practices unless this is done.

Collaboration, reflection and documentation

It is both surprising and yet unsurprising how frequently I meet staff teams who are working with a person providing serious challenges, yet they do not carry out the most basically useful record keeping on this aspect of their work. One team were in the slough of despair, with very poor morale. They did have some desultory documentation from which it was possible to piece together some kind of picture about what they had been doing. Having done that, it seemed possible that there had actually been a big improvement in the person's behaviour during the recent months, perhaps 20 per cent less incidents, but the staff hadn't noticed. They should have been doing 'high fives' in the staff room. However, since they did not keep records with any great thoroughness, nor collate them effectively, they were not even able to reward themselves with this information.

If a person's behaviour improves in the order of only five per cent less incidents over a month or two, that is positive information really worth having. However, a five per cent improvement is not the sort of figure that can be subjectively assessed. ('I dunno, what do you think Mary, do you think he's got better lately?') This can only be done systematically.

Acquiring a continuous picture about whether there are more or less incidents occurring is one of the most obvious pieces of record keeping to carry out. It will usually need to go further than that of course. It is important to have perspectives on whether the reduction of incidents is due to the person's improving state or the staff's improving defusing abilities. Some of the contributors document the value of recordings which helped identify triggers to incidents and describe antecedents. Several of them describe the amount of effort which goes into positively evaluating, looking to identify and record staff technique which worked, and the formative experience for staff of sitting together and doing this. There is an atmosphere that the writers enjoyed this aspect of their work, particularly the collaboration with colleagues that it engendered and the sense of positive purposefulness arising during discussion and reflection.

Creating a record-keeping system which will give the information necessary can be somewhat difficult, but it is not an intensely demanding intellectual exercise. The really difficult aspect of record keeping seems to be being motivated to do it. Many things can be barriers, and the amount of stress that staff can be under and the extent to which they may be overwhelmed by their working circumstances is one of them. In recent years, employers have shown more of a tendency to compel staff to carry out documentation, and I applaud the message sent by their efforts. However, I have a preference for employers attempting to do more to motivate staff to achieve the enjoyment and job satisfaction from documentation which is clear in the work of the staff writing here.

Teamwork and team practices

Occasionally I meet staff groups who do not have good teamwork and do not look likely to achieve it. I feel sad for the people with learning difficulties they are serving, but I feel sad for the staff too as they are missing out on one of the best rewards their work has to offer. There are usually two main factors in a lack of teamwork. One factor is the sheer duress of the job: staff having too much to do, a timetable that is too intense, too many expectations about what they will achieve, no time being made available to them for thought, discussion and collaboration with others. The other factor is usually the complex dynamics of the different personalities which make up the group. One thing is clear – a lack of teamwork is likely to be a prime environmental factor in the production of challenging behaviour by service-users (see Figure 1.3, 'All communication difficulties').

There is much evidence of good and enjoyable teamwork in this book, and Chapter 9 contains some pointers to elements of good teamwork during incidents of challenging behaviour. However, I fear that the contributors may not help the staff groups who fall into the description above, since it can be difficult to achieve effective teamworking by reading a book, particularly with regard to overcoming the complex dynamics of a group of personalities. Perhaps there is one major piece of advice clear from the work documented here. Teamwork does not happen accidentally because nice people find themselves in the same place. The staff writing here show the extent to which they looked each other in the eyes and talked. Sometimes that talking needs to be gritty and direct and this can be a hard thing to do. There is, however, no substitute for it. There is thus much advice about the hard work necessary to achieve teamwork, including the preparedness to have the difficult discussions.

Constant thought on balancing service-users' rights with staff duty of care

This can be one of the most complex aspects of the job facing staff I meet. It concerns issues unlikely ever to be completely resolved. However, it will aid the effectiveness of staff teams if they have regular discussion of this aspect of their philosophy. Ideally, these discussion will help them to know each other's individual attitudes and arrive at some sort of common attitude which should be borne out and be visible in their moment-by-moment working practices. The basic question is: to what extent do service-users have a right to do what they wish and to what extent do staff have a duty to compel them to do what they wish?

In adult services, the issue is a little easier for staff than in schools. There is, or there should be, some sort of general appreciation that the service-users are citizens with the same rights over their lives as all other citizens. That does not mean that staff should instantly accept all of the person's preferences for behaviour and lifestyle. It is an unavoidable duty of staff to make judgements and decisions on behalf of people as to what is in their best interests. This is particularly the case if one person's preferences infringes another person's free-doms or lifestyle or if the person's preferences are unhealthy or hazardous for her/himself. This usually involves staff in a fair amount of legitimate 'goal-blocking' – preventing people from doing things that they wish to do. It is also the duty of staff to make general decisions about what the person may best learn to enhance the person's quality of life, and to pursue these aims with energy.

However, the recognition of the person's rights as a citizen should affect the staff behaviour in pursuing the aims. Simply because staff have these duties of care should not imply that the authority they then have legitimises unjustly forceful behaviour to achieve the aims. Staff should show determination, but they should be determined to motivate, to achieve participation and co-operation, to demonstrate to the service-user the worth of what they are offering. Any goal-blocking, coercion or forceful intervention should be carried out well but with reluctance, and the staff should show a clear respect for the person's basic rights in a style which avoids a sense of dominance while still being effective.

The situation is only slightly different in schools, though the issue of children's rights and teachers' duties can seem more complex and more pressing. Children's rights may be seen to include less immediate freedoms, for good reasons. In law they *must* be at school, and teachers correspondingly have more duties – they *must* teach them. The law reflects society's view of what is seen as children's needs, including the security of adult direction and protection. Few people would disagree with the correctness of this view of children's rights. However, I think that the same points outlined above about staff behaviour can still apply. Simply because children must be there, does this imply that they must comply at all times? No successful teacher I meet believes that children must simply comply at all times and this attitude is reflected in a positive style of managing behaviour. The best mainstream practice sees schools gradually handing over responsibility for behaviour to pupils as they grow older. Thus, all nursery age children need to be protected and directed more than older children in primary schools or secondary schools, where there is an assumption that pupils gradually take more responsibility for their lives. Young people with learning difficulties and challenging behaviour need more protection and direction than their mainstream peers, but they have the right to be treated according to the same principles.

For instance, if Rosemary Hawkins or Bernard Emblem and staff held the absolute view that it is the teacher's job to give orders and the children's job simply to comply, they would probably let themselves into a great deal of stress and difficulty with some young people who find it difficult even to sit down for any length of time. They do fully recognise, however, that it is their job to work endlessly at helping their pupils to learn the things that they want them to do, such as sitting down. By having a realistic and relaxed attitude to the children's ability to comply in the short term, they open themselves up to being flexible and creative in achieving their goals. This may sound like an obvious and logical argument, but it is possible to meet members of staff in all services whose practice is limited and lacks creativity because of their insistence on immediate compliance and their inability to accept 'no' temporarily. They tend to experience some needlessly confrontational situations.

Naturally, doing things that one does not want to do can be a healthy experience for all people occasionally and we all endure it sometimes in various ways. One of the considerations that we must bring to this work however, is judgements about whether a person's major experience of life is like this. This can occur when there is a wide gap or mismatch between any rigidity of what is on offer in a service provision and the nature of a person's abilities, understandings and needs. One of

13

the results of this mismatch between the service and the person can be some behaviour which is described as 'challenging'.

Teachers in schools for pupils with severe learning difficulties can be particularly vexed by this issue. They are presented with the apparently conflicting demands of the National Curriculum attainments for each pupil, and the need to design for many pupils a 'personal' curriculum, much of which may seem to fall outside the National Curriculum programmes of study. Many severe learning difficulties (SLD) teachers and schools have been wonderfully creative and flexible in achieving the necessary balances on this issue, welcoming the broadening of what schools must offer, but at the same time not placing the onus on the pupil to fit into it. They deliver an imaginative and flexible National Curriculum together with a wholesome personal curriculum focusing on matters such as communicating and relating. The School Curriculum and Assessment Authority also responded to the issue, and their document (SCAA 1996) is essential reading for teachers (and inspectors) working with pupils with the more severe learning difficulties who are still troubled by the issue.

As has been implied in this discussion, there is not a formula for getting this whole issue 'right'. The keyword I think is in the title to the section – 'balance'. The balancing act should be ongoing and constantly under review and it is likely to be a different balancing act for different pupils or adult clients – the enormous variation of ability likely in any group of people with learning difficulties makes this differentiation a practical necessity. Furthermore, it is a good idea for staff always to be dissatisfied with the balance they are working with and discuss it frequently.

Interest and enjoyment

It would be easy to pass over the sensation arising out of the accounts in this book that the staff thoroughly enjoy their work. This does not mean by any stretch of the imagination that every moment of every day is a hoot for them, but that they like and respect the person they are helping, they find intellectual enjoyment and fulfilment, and they probably have plenty of fun with service-users and other staff. Helping a person who is being challenging to learn more about enjoying life is likely to address some significant personal factors in that person's challenging behaviour. It is difficult for staff who are not finding the work enjoyable to achieve this.

Geraint Ephraim's enjoyment (Chapter 12) of all aspects of what he does is evident in the way he writes about it. I know for certain that he is infectious with this attitude, looking to pass some of it on to all front-line staff with whom he collaborates. The stresses of work can make it easy for staff to forget this aspect of it, but anyone who is reading these words is surely doing so because they find interest and enjoyment in their work. The most difficult periods of the work are most definitely the time to make an effort to remember this.

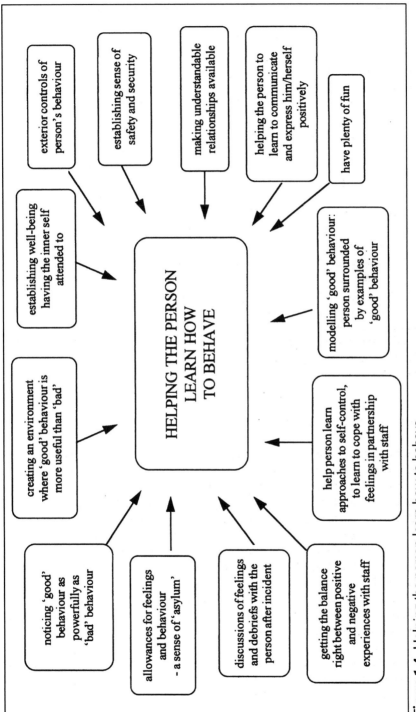

Figure 1.4 Helping the person learn how to behave

15

Resolution – help the person learn how to behave

Another way of viewing the practical complexities of the work of the contributors to this book is set out in Figure 1.4. It is an attempt at a visual 'map' of an ecological approach to helping a person with challenging behaviour. The work here is focused on a concept of 'helping the person learn how to behave'. The smaller boxes display examples of the things the staff need to do in the environment around the person and with the person, to the person.

'Helping the person learn how to behave' is a phrase borrowed and modified from Leach (1977). She was attempting to point out that nurturing children who have good behaviour involved an extensive and positive concept of 'showing children how to behave', involving more than crude notions of control and discipline. That intention is here too, but it is worth stressing that staff use of exterior controls of a person's behaviour does appear as one of the boxes. The issue is, to borrow a phrase from Bernie Hunt (Chapter 6), that having exterior controls such as clear boundaries is an aspect of the way that they work, but it is not a definition of it.

'Helping the person learn how to behave' is a more open, positive and far-reaching concept than more often seen phrases such as 'dealing with' or 'overcoming' challenging behaviour. Use of it as a working concept can help to open up staff to the variety of measures that need to be taken to help the person and the need to do more than simply focus on the removal of the behaviour.

References

Clements, J. (1997) 'Sustaining a cognitive psychology for people with learning disabilities', in Stenfert Kroese, B., Dagnan, D., Loumidis, K. (eds) *Cognitive Behaviour Therapy for People with Learning Disabilities*. London: Routledge.

Harris, J. and Hewett, D. (1996) *Positive Approaches to Challenging Behaviours*. Kidderminster: First Draft Publications (BILD).

Leach, P. (1977) *Baby and Child*. Harmondsworth: Penguin.

Nind, M. and Hewett, D. (1994) *Access to Communication: Developing the Basics of Communication with People with Severe Learning Difficulties Through Intensive Interaction*. London: David Fulton Publishers.

SCAA (1996) *Planning the Curriculum for Pupils with Profound and Multiple Learning Difficulties*. London: SCAA.

Stenfert Kroese, B. (1997) 'Cognitive-behaviour therapy for people with learning disabilities: conceptual and contextual issues', in Stenfert Kroese, B., Dagnan, D., Loumidis, K. (eds) *Cognitive Behaviour Therapy for People with Learning Disabilities*. London: Routledge.

Chapter 2

Positive incident management – insights from staff involved and issues for the organisation

Martin Bertulis, Paul Norton, Paul Jones,
Carol Cadwallader, Pam Grounds and Steve McGreevy

Introduction

The following chapter describes positive, interactive approaches used with a student who presents severely challenging and violent behaviours, sometimes without apparent cause or warning. Brief descriptions will be presented about the school, the students concerned, the setting and the staff support system.

The main focus of the chapter is about five cases of incident management from the perspective of five different carers and educators. Sometimes the member of staff is able to show the process of thinking and feeling as they deal with the incident. In others, members of staff are more reactive having to cope with the unexpected, often 'thinking on their feet' and having to 'go with it'. Names have been changed to protect each individual's confidentiality.

The school

Womaston School was set up by MacIntyre Care in 1986 to serve up to 23 children and young people with severe learning disabilities between the ages of 7 and 19. The youngsters all exhibit challenging behaviours including violence and self injury and often show evidence of autism or emotional disturbance.

A common thread for most of the students is that they cannot live at home and/or that school services have broken down. In several cases local services have not met their needs despite valiant, well-intentioned and skilled intervention. In many cases the 24-hour consistency of approach at the school has helped almost every student to repair themselves and to develop after several years of major trauma.

There have been three students in the 11-year history of the school who we have had to exclude. In each case the frequency of violent behaviour exhibited by each person had reduced or stayed the same but the intensity had grown, often linked to physical stature or mental health issues, requiring physical interventions incompatible with the status of the school or the training of the staff. Sometimes we are limited as a school because the time required to make real change may be too great as some students are referred at age 15–16 years and need to leave in their 19th year. Some students will leave the school positively at 19, where student, staff and family have learned to manage difficult behaviours without changing underlying behaviour, an achievement which should be acknowledged and celebrated. The school is therefore based on a 52-week flexible residential model to enable optimum family contact.

The school employs positive approaches building on strengths and aptitudes to open more appropriate channels of communication and achievement for each student. The school has developed an empathic approach attempting to find the meaning to behaviour and to understand the feelings evoked by students. The school uses aspects of behavioural approaches, *Gentle Teaching* (McGee *et al.* 1987), therapeutic interventions and Intensive Interaction (Nind and Hewett, 1994). Communication and personal and social education underpin and link all aspects of the curriculum for each student. A simple way to describe the approach might be that we help the student to change inside by making many changes to the outside.

The student

Trevor is a tall, agile teenager who functions at a severe learning disability level and exhibits behaviours which severely challenge. His behaviour also shows many features consistent with some degree of autism. He can also be a friendly, sociable young man who enjoys interacting with others, usually on his terms.

Trevor vocalises, sometimes alarmingly, but doesn't use words. He uses a few Makaton signs consistently but his main means of communication is by taking a person's hand to do something. It becomes apparent that he also communicates through eye contact, facial expression and the initiation of interactive games including chase. It is extremely difficult to establish what Trevor understands and how he sees the world. It is easy to misconstrue the apparent meaning of a behaviour and to view it purely in bullying or dominating terms. Trevor evokes a range of powerful feelings and emotions in the people he encounters. When being objective this is easily understood since the behaviours he exhibits can be violent, intrusive, unexpected, appearing from nowhere and potentially dangerous to fellow students and members of staff.

Trevor appears to make attempts to control the environment and will take action if that control is threatened or routine disrupted. The resulting behaviours include pushing, pinching, thumping, slapping, pulling hair, breaking spectacles, ripping clothes and head butting. Trevor also injures himself by biting himself and hitting his head on windows, or slapping his own head.

By careful management and a constant quest to understand Trevor's world, Trevor has a good quality of life and presents as a relatively happy, although somewhat anxious, young man for much of the time.

An excerpt from Trevor's profile gives information to staff about the student with some explanation, background and some practical guidance:

Trevor does not have any speech. He is a very independent-minded young man and likes to do things for himself. He is autistic and does not really understand about communication; that he needs to, or that he can. Rather than ask for something, Trevor would prefer to do everything for himself.

We must help Trevor to understand this 'necessity to communicate' and build it into his everyday life. Therefore at all times when Trevor wants something we must help him to demonstrate this in some way, e.g. by signing or pointing or tapping a picture. At present Trevor will take you by the hand to get you to do something or take keys to get into the cupboard for something. We must model forms of communication for Trevor to copy and then adopt, i.e.:

(a) If he wants an object he should be asked to sign 'a key' or 'more' or 'biscuit'. Very often he will need to copy the sign, occasionally he will sign without staff having to model it, but generally he does not sign spontaneously as yet, but has to be asked to sign.

(b) Trevor does not use pointing to communicate. Staff must model pointing either in a general way (the direction) or to a picture or object to make a choice or to make his needs known. Staff must then encourage Trevor to point also.

Trevor can be mischievous and full of fun. He enjoys physical games but only on his terms, and he prefers to instigate these. Trevor uses touch games to let you know how things are. By carefully matching his touch (usually on hands and arms) a physical conversation can take place. This is also instigated by Trevor in a restoration phase after an incident. Members of staff need to learn to listen to and read these touch sequences. As he gains trust in the staff member he is willing to tolerate more play and fun type interactions that are instigated by that member of staff. Trevor requires time to get to know new staff. Do not expect him to accept you or comply with your requests straight away. He is shy and cautious.

In class Trevor can be quite noisy. He makes short loud low sounds and he quite enjoys you copying these. He will also touch and give good eye contact and 'nuzzle up' to staff sitting next to him. He enjoys being talked to and he responds by smiling or laughing and other facial expressions. If he is unsure, he tends to half close his eyes as if to shut you out.

Trevor understands a lot in context. Often we may be discussing the day's activities and will tell Trevor that later he will be going on the bus and when it is time he is packed up and waiting to go.

However it is possible to overestimate Trevor's level of understanding. He understands a lot through routines. At times the world must seem a frightening and unpredictable environment to Trevor.

If Trevor is upset or anxious about anything he will hit out, scratch, throw items or will attack other students. On these occasions he responds to a strong, firm approach, a firm 'Stop that' or 'No Trevor'. Due to his difficulties in communicating he cannot explain to us why he is upset. He does not want to behave inappropriately and he needs a lot of reassurance at these times.

The setting

Trevor lives with four other young men in a residential unit on the school campus. He has his own bedroom which he uses very appropriately and it clearly serves the purpose of being a place of safety and security. This place of safety is an essential part of Trevor's and our strategy in managing his difficult behaviour.

Trevor goes to school on the same campus currently with the same young men who share a house with him. Some activities are set up so that students from different houses and classes can join together.

The staff from the residential unit also spend time in the classrooms during education time and the teacher and education-based RSWs (residential support workers) are attached to the house. This minimises the number of direct carers and educators linked to each individual.

The school is set in a rural location in 20 acres of grounds. The nearest small towns of Presteigne and Kington are 5 miles away and the larger towns of Llandrindod Wells, Hereford and Shrewsbury are 20, 25 and 40 miles away, respectively.

The campus gives physical space to all in a relatively safe setting. Additionally, the way the school works aims to give people space to develop emotionally and intellectually. It would be easy to confuse this at first sight with the old concept of asylum where people were locked away and in many ways 'out of sight out of mind'.

I am beginning to use the concept of 'positive asylum' to differentiate what we do from previous negative connotations. Briefly, I am talking about a place where a person is able to develop safety from the outside and from within, where people are given appropriate time and space and are accepted for who they are, their behaviour being listened to but not defining the person. This ethos can occur in every setting be it rural or urban. In many ways it is defined by the attitudes, systems and ethos of an establishment. We constantly have the internal debate about how to provide a quality environment without locking everything up and bolting down furniture. There is no magical answer but by keeping the debate alive we are less likely to fall into very unreal and stagnant work practice.

The school has to prepare students to leave, which puts a natural developmental onus into all we do. Being more specific about Trevor, it becomes clear that he has more opportunity for moving about the campus with staff at an appropriate distance. In an urban environment he would always need two people available with one person at his side. One of the plans for Trevor is for him to generalise his confidence on a campus setting to known and unknown urban environments. It is also part of our job to help Trevor to understand and tell us in some way about the kind of environment he would like to live in. This is a real challenge but is a key task. A final general observation about the rural setting is that in this fast moving crowded world physical space is an important amenity.

Planning the programme

The overall plans for each student begin to evolve at the assessment stage where information is given by parents, carers and authority representatives. The 'Can I envisage X living at Womaston?' question begins to be asked and answered from the parents first contact with the school. Once placement is agreed, objectives are set by reference to the educational statement of special needs and the care plan.

The school actively welcomes outreach support during the students move to the school by carers or parents who can help the individual and the school staff to understand each other. It is often apparently small details which can 'derail' a move – a special night-time drink, a way of saying something, music on or off in the bedroom when settling at night.

Given that at least 15 people will be directly involved in an individual's care and education, it is essential that clear and regular communication takes place. The main vehicles for this are: the core group meeting approximately monthly where the teacher, key worker and senior staff review the progress of the individual to modify and set new targets (or to start again!) and weekly house meetings which include education input, exchange of information and discussion of weekly fine tuning around each student.

After the initial six months there is a six-monthly individual plan/individual education plan (IP/IEP) care review to include parents, authority representatives and the student where possible to review the previous six months and to set new target goals (see Figure 2.1).

Systems, training and support

Enabling a team of about 15 people to work with a complex person like Trevor presents real challenges both individually and for an organisation. Guidelines are important for all staff who work with Trevor – they cannot work in a vacuum. However the guidelines must take account of the need to be consistent with Trevor, but this doesn't mean that all staff should do exactly the same thing. Policy and guidance need to be regularly updated and modified, often quite subtly. These changes need to be communicated and monitored to and by all of the staff team.

The regular core group and weekly house meetings are the working meetings which plan, develop, monitor and evaluate the service experienced by Trevor. It is here that guidelines will be written and amended. As previously implied, getting it down on paper is difficult and it never tells the complete story. Therefore the use of house meetings and handovers regularly allows us to talk around and about the guidelines to give them life.

The school is developing practice supervision. A training forum to present and reflect upon our practice with students and the meaning of behaviours. This is a multidisciplinary and cross-site training which helps us to learn from experience and link theory with practice.

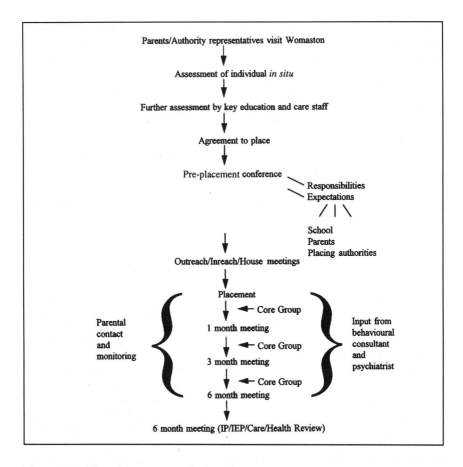

Figure 2.1 The placement and planning process

Training is provided externally and internally in a variety of approaches. In the case of Trevor intensive interaction and gentle teaching are useful as direct tools but they also help to underline appropriate attitudes. For helping Trevor, training about autism has also been developed internally, with regular use of outside training in working with autism. Throughout this training much emphasis is placed on empathic approaches. Clearly incidents will occur, and the management of these incidents is carefully thought about. Physical training is given alongside work on low arousal approaches, diffusion and resolution.

Staff are often left feeling shocked, angry, upset and guilty, and are offered an immediate debriefing session. Sometimes a second debrief follows if further issues are raised which cannot, or should not, be discussed immediately after an incident. There may be aspects of practice in staff behaviour which can be improved. Informing and teaching someone about this is better done when feelings and adrenalin are back to normal levels.

There are times when the traumatic event touches an issue which needs external support. In these cases external counselling is provided by the general practitioner of the member of staff or by private external counselling paid for by the school; these events rarely happen. It probably works a little like insurance – if you have it available you don't always need it, and vice versa!

The following are real examples of situations and how they were dealt with by Trevor and the members of staff around him. They are not all examples of 'perfect practice'. In some cases, on reflection, parts of the incident may have been handled differently. However, in a real and dynamic setting much learning takes place during or after incidents even when they 'go wrong'. This learning helps to inform us for the next difficult incident.

The members of staff have written the accounts from a very personal perspective, and I provide commentaries after each one to highlight points which seem to be important.

Case study 1 – Paul Norton (acting head of home)

It may be useful to describe the layout of the house. It is built on three levels: ground floor – kitchen, living areas and garden; upper floor – bedrooms and bathrooms; middle level – half way between the front door and the sleep-in-room/office, with a doorway to the stairs. The bulk of my administration work is done in the sleep-in-room/office in the house.

When a violent incident occurs I first know about it when there is an urgent shout for help or I am called by name. My first thoughts are: Who is involved?; Is anyone hurt?; Where are they?; What can I do? My priority is to ensure that everyone is safe, both students and staff. My aim then is to get any staff who are hurt or stressed away from the situation to get help. I also direct other staff to take other students who would be at risk away from the situation. Then, after ensuring that everyone is safe I turn my attention to the student who is behaving aggressively (although sometimes dealing with the violent student may have to be the main priority to prevent further injury). In dealing with the student I try to be non-confrontational, keeping my hands down, speaking calmly and clearly, not using too many words. I try to reassure the student, encourage him to sit down or go to his room where we can be quiet together, or go to his room where he can be as noisy and jump around as much as he likes, as long as he stays there. Going and staying in his room, followed by settling in his favourite chair are good signs!

One particular incident started in the way I've described. I was working in the office when I heard an urgent call for help. I grabbed my keys and ran to the door, but I didn't know where the incident was occurring. It was lunch time and my first reaction was to go downstairs. I soon discovered the incident had occurred on the upstairs landing.

I found Carol sitting on the floor of the landing, Debbie was with her fending off blows from Trevor and protecting Carol. I immediately got Trevor's attention by calling his name and telling him very firmly to go to his room. I needed to 'stand up' to Trevor in a calm firm but non-aggressive manner. I assumed that my body language was saying, 'Listen to me, you need to do this', and I used direct eye contact to establish the point. He did go to his room, and I was able to praise him for being there. Carol and Debbie moved to the adjacent bathroom.

While Trevor stayed in his bedroom, I instructed two other staff to lock themselves in the sitting room (access to garden) to ensure the safety of themselves and two students who were also in the house. When I returned to Trevor he had pulled down the curtains in his room and thrown them downstairs. He ran into the dining room and pulled those curtains down too. I directed Trevor back to his room again and he ran towards me and scratched my hands and grabbed my arm, bruising it, then he ran to his room. He was very noisy in his room but for the moment stayed there.

I spoke to Carol and Debbie in the bathroom and got them to go downstairs to the office where they would be safe. I then remained with Trevor in the safe space that had been created for him: he had his room, two bathrooms, landings and stairs, dining room and downstairs toilet in which he could move with minimal interaction from me. I gave him as much space as I could. During this time (10–15 min) I reassured him as often as I felt appropriate. He remained in quite an agitated state, at one point taking off his shirt and throwing it downstairs. I asked him to put on another and he used my keys to do that, then he remained in his room. He still remained in his room most of the time and his agitation appeared to be decreasing. Shortly afterwards two staff from the house where Trevor used to live came to give their support and helped Trevor to calm down.

During the incident I'm not sure that I thought about how scared I was. Safety of others and Trevor were the overriding thoughts. I did not neglect my own safety either, but used the skills that I have gained from six years of experience in this field and the training I have received.

I am aware of a difficult balance needed in managing the incident I needed to be clear and in control without intimidating or frightening Trevor. He seems to need people that can 'stand up to him in a caring way'.

On reflection I was scared. Trevor is taller, stronger, more supple and faster than I am and was a very real threat. He had previously broken two staff members' noses when agitated. But in creating a safe space for Trevor and myself I was able to give minimalist interaction and maximum space for him to work out his anger in his own way. The ethos of my intervention was to sort out the situation – not to punish or lay blame on anyone.

Afterwards I discovered that Trevor had pushed Carol against the wall momentarily knocking her out. Senior staff were available to debrief all staff involved, and staff from another house took Carol to the local hospital to be checked over.

The reasons why the incident occurred when it did are not clear, but some possibilities could be that:

- Trevor insists on his key being in his bedroom door. He had been out swimming and during this time another student had meddled with his key. It had been placed in the office with the intention of replacing it just before he returned. This wasn't done, so when Trevor came back the key was not there, which would have made him anxious.
- He also was not able to put his coat away by himself when he returned (a staff member offered to do it).
- He may have been particularly anxious that week because it was half term from school so he did not have regular contact with his teacher and education-based RSW. He has an excellent relationship with the education-based RSW.

I had, at the time, responsibility for the day to day functioning of the house which included the writing of rotas and planning the combination of staff on shift. Trevor had moved to the house three weeks previously from another house on site and was still coming to terms with his new environment and staff group. He appears to respond better to male staff rather than female staff, so in planning the rota I needed to take this into account, as well as ensuring staff who had a good relationship with Trevor were also on shift. We had received a good handover for Trevor with staff from his old house working alongside the house staff for a week and then staff being on call should we need them. In school Trevor remained in the same classroom with a familiar teacher and education-based RSW, so only his home life changed.

Commentary on – case study 1 Martin Bertulis

In case study 1, Paul eloquently describes some of the thoughts, feelings and issues experienced by senior staff who intervened to help to restore equilibrium with students and staff. It is not always clear why an incident has occurred, which means that the member of staff is in the dark and rapidly needs to see, hear and feel what is going on. This is a teamwork issue where information can be passed by looks, nods and few words. Of course sometimes there is less information available and the term 'informed flying by the seat of your pants' comes to mind.

Initial management is essential in stopping the spiral of dangerous behaviour. Once this is achieved then careful de-escalation and space-giving techniques are used.

Debriefing other students who may have witnessed some or all of the incident is important. These students need to know that everything has been resolved. They also may need to vent their feelings appropriately. We often see a series of incidents occurring where we perceive that the initial cause may have been about another student's difficulty much earlier in the day. I think that we need to do more to help the onlookers/by standers in this kind of incident. The first step is to recognise that it needs to be done. A final thought on this case is about making the intervention helpful to both staff and students and not undermining the people involved in the incident. We spend a lot of time developing a culture which says:

- It is OK to ask for help – you don't lose face.
- It is OK to offer support at any time, preferably before something happens. In fact it is clear that a change of face is a simple but very potent way of defusing many inflamed situations. We also need to pay attention to situations which keep occurring between specific staff and students. This often gives us a lot of very useful information to work with.

Case study 2 – Paul Jones (education-based RSW)

Trevor had to move house four weeks before this incident. He did not understand the reasons why he was moved and was still insecure about his peers and immediate surroundings. It was first thing Monday morning after half-term break. On arrival at the house I was greeted by an immediate realisation that Trevor was agitated and very upset. He was wailing very loudly, running up and down the stairs, often missing the last four steps and almost leaping, and slamming doors.

He followed me down a flight of approximately four steps between the kitchen and the lounge. Here we were face to face giving each other eye contact. Trevor was crying and rocking from side to side and jumping up and down. I asked Trevor in a calm voice 'What is the matter? Calm down Trevor'. At this point Trevor began pinching at both of my arms and hitting out, and I received scratches to the back of my hands. I was aware of the space between Trevor and myself at that point because of the possibility that I could receive a head butt.

After having a well-earned and relaxing week off, my feelings on returning back to an incident of this magnitude certainly made my adrenalin flow. I remember vividly my left knee shaking uncontrollably and thinking to myself 'On no, I don't need this shit!'

Another member of staff appeared by my side and I was able to unlock the door leading to the garden where Trevor followed. He then jumped over the fence and ran up the drive wailing and crying.

I knew that Trevor needs space after an incident and that he runs away until calm and then comes back – up to now at least. I knew that I had to keep my distance as crowding him would have heightened his state of arousal. This was difficult because Trevor was heading towards the road. I'm responsible and yet I can't get too close. Why me? I was about 200 yards away at first keeping Trevor in sight. A colleague alerted management to send a car round to keep tabs on us and I was given an aid call to get help if needed. I could tell by the way that he was wailing less that he was calming down. I edged closer little by little. He was still going away from the school on the road but slower now. He usually turns round of his own accord although usually much earlier! He turned round and began to walk back and I closed in even more. By the time he got back to the car park at the school we were walking together. I was quietly commenting that he was calmer, 'What are you like Trevor!' 'Glad you're calm'. Although close, we were still distanced. He was looking away and his eyes were squinting at times. I opened the door of his house and he went up to his room. He remained based in there all morning, although he popped out occasionally. Staying in the room and making the odd foray out of it is a good sign. He was outwardly calm by lunchtime. However, in hindsight it took us a few months to become really close again.

This incident happened several months ago and nothing on this scale has happened since. I'm still learning about Trevor. One of the teachers at the school put it really well, 'Working with Trevor is like playing a musical instrument'. I suppose that means that you may have all the training and programmes sorted out (the notes) but you still need to feel the instrument to play the music.

Commentary on case study 2 – Martin Bertulis

Trevor's guidelines note that 'Trevor calms more quickly when given his own space . . . this includes his bedroom, the garden, and his seat in the lounge'. His own space does not usually include the public highway with all its inherent dangers. It is clear that physical intervention would have been physically dangerous and damaging to relationships between Trevor and members of staff. Of course it would have been an option if the road had been very busy and the student was running down the middle of it. Additional staffing would have been summoned to help here.

This case shows very careful reaction and management to a potentially life-threatening situation. Careful observation skills were used which allowed the member of staff to gradually help Trevor to regain a sense of equilibrium. The member of staff remembered one of the basics in management guidelines 'at any stage when Trevor complies with your request praise him for this'.

Paul notes that 'a person appeared by my side'. This underlines the important teamwork which is needed here. With Trevor it is usually clear if there is a problem. This is not always the case, and other techniques may be used – a pager system which summons support or well chosen key words can signify 'Help now!' without escalating the situation. Ideally an extra person can arrive on the scene before an incident happens – the new face can be a good distracter and a calming influence. We also know well that if two or three big men arrive at speed it can only mean one thing!

Case study 3 – Pam Grounds (teacher)

Trevor's entry into the classroom often gives me plenty of clues about how he is feeling that day: how he opens the door (tentatively or pushed strongly on its hinges); how fast he moves to his seat; the quality of his noise making; whether he gives eye contact; how well he tolerates his peers – if he pushes them out of the way gently or more roughly; how near he will tolerate my sitting by him; if he responds to a 'Hello' or a touch; how mobile he is when sat down – sometimes he sways gently and moves his hands rhythmically, at other times he sits very still. Tuning in to Trevor takes time and needs active discussion with other staff in handovers, core groups and team days to get the message across. It is hard. Yet there is no firm rule. He can be tense and quiet, but he can also be tense and noisy. Sometimes he gives lots of eye contact, but this can mean he is in a more heightened state than if he shifts his gaze uneasily. I do know that he gets reassurance from my acknowledgement of his presence. I try to be warm but light in my greetings. He also gains reassurance from following the general routine. Our communication sessions are boisterous, fun-type sessions. Trevor enjoys rolling a huge jingle ball across the table to people and our singing of noisy songs that include his name. These sessions can go really well or really badly. When it goes well I really feel close to Trevor and to other students. He is also very aware of who else is in the classroom and who may be missing.

That morning I was without my classroom assistant. The other staff with me were fairly new but appeared confident with Trevor. The communication session had been successful and Trevor was allowed to return to his favourite activity – cutting up pieces of paper very small and collecting the bits in a tub.

Another student was needing attention and I was going to have to leave the room with him. I explained to the RSW the task Trevor could be asked to do when he was ready and gave him the equipment (picture matching), but I also said that if Trevor did not want to do it that was fine. I sensed Trevor was not totally calm because of the unfamiliar staff, but he did not seem too anxious and the staff reassured me that he had worked with Trevor a lot in the house and had no worries.

I returned to class about 5–10 minutes later. The RSW explained that Trevor had complied with his request, tidied the cutting away and started the activity, but had abruptly left his seat, pushed another student over off his chair and then pushed the RSW over. Both staff were shocked and Trevor was very tense. As this was being explained I sat near Trevor. I sensed he was on the point of getting up again. As he made to move I said a strong 'No Trevor', followed by 'It's alright Trevor'. Trevor sat down again but he was clutching the table and was very wary. I stroked his arm to try and reassure. I felt he was going to jump up and either push or hit or throw something at any minute.

He stopped tolerating my stroke and began to pinch my arm and scratch my hand. But this was not as severe as he can do, the quality of his scratching is very indicative of how uneasy he is – sometimes he will just turn his fingers to press his nails against the back of your hand just letting you know things are not OK, but when really aroused he seems to slash. This pressure was in between the two. I reacted to the scratching, said a further 'No Trevor' and withdrew a little.

A short interval; busying myself with boxes and pictures on the table. I felt we needed a change of mood. Apart from the student who had been out of the room with me who seemed oblivious to the tension in the room, all attention was on Trevor, although I was sitting side on and not facing him. This is necessary because it seems important to be 'with' him and not 'against' him. I can work in parallel to him not opposite him.

I turned to him and said briskly, 'Right Trevor, you can get your cutting out now'. To my relief he did so and picked up his box with his paper and scissors and started arranging things in front of him.

I spoke quietly to the other RSWs to take the other two students out of the room and I sat with Trevor avoiding eye contact but singing and talking to myself pretending to be busy with things on the table and pretending to be calm. Gradually Trevor relaxed and so did I.

Had this not worked, i.e. Trevor had not taken up his cutting, I felt Trevor would have possibly left the classroom, which is fine; it is policy to give Trevor space. However, I wanted to contain him if possible because I was aware that he could have done some damage on the way out had he left in a heightened frame of mind (pushing or hitting people and possibly meeting unaware or vulnerable people outside).

Commentary on case study 3 – Martin Bertulis

On the face of it this case illustrates how dependent Trevor is on people being in the right place at the right time. Both the teacher and education-based RSW were not present in the room for a short time.

The incident was quickly defused and calmness restored. I am particularly impressed by the awareness of those small nuances of behaviour which can say so much (the quality of the scratching), the awareness of seating position (side on) and the timing of changing the activity. A lot of proactive thought and mood matching was going on to ensure everyone's physical and emotional safety.

I am aware that Pam is able to work in a very sensitive and empathic manner. She talks about 'tuning-in' – this takes skill, experience, and an appropriate attitude which really believes in listening to behaviour rather than approaching the situation in a judgemental manner.

Pam is a teacher and has a clear role in demonstrating and writing down the approaches. It would be interesting to find out if the approach can be deconstructed and taught to other members of staff. We endeavour to do this with values-based training, empathic work, practise supervision and the use of the core team meetings. I do sometimes wonder how much of the approach can be learnt by training and how much is based on the existing inner resources of the individual member of staff. It would be complacent to imagine that our training hits the mark every time, although conversely it clearly does hit the mark sometimes!

Case study 4 – Carol Cadwallader (RSW grade 3)

Description of what was taking place:

Trevor had led me to the lounge and took me to the television cabinet. He then took my keys from me and started to open the cabinet. Then Trevor went and sat down. I tried to get the TV to work but it would not. I then remembered that we had turned the power off (this was due to a resident urinating on the switches in his room and we were waiting for maintenance to attend to the switches). I said to Trevor that I was going to the office to put the power on. As I went up the stairs to the office Trevor thumped me on the back. I turned to tell Trevor to 'Stop', when he slapped my face taking my glasses at the same time breaking them in half. I said to Trevor 'Go to your room' but he pushed me hard and I went up against the wall. I then shouted for assistance from other staff. Trevor continued to try and hit me and I put my arms up to protect my head and tried to ward off the blows. I called for help, Stuart, another member of staff came to my assistance and Trevor went to his room. Part of Trevor's procedures after incidents are to give him plenty of space and time on his own and for a second person to be there. Sometimes a change of face or a second person is enough to change things with no further action needed.

Thoughts, feelings, fears and anxieties

With the first thump I thought 'What the heck?', then with the slap I thought Trevor was angry due to his body language and noise he was making. I felt very frightened when he pushed me against the wall and I had to defend myself. I put my hands across my face in a textbook manner. However I think I did this by reflex rather than training. It also seemed an eternity before assistance came but it must have been only a minute or so.

The whole incident lasted 10 to 15 minutes. I kept thinking 'keep calm, do not shout and be careful with eye contact', but it is very difficult when you have somebody coming at you all the time and you feel there is no way out of it. Losing my glasses leaves me even more vulnerable and defenceless. I use contact lenses now and so feel more confident. Often it is possible to help Trevor out and defuse the incident by asking him to go to his room, his calming space or to jolly him out of it – 'Come on, Trevor pack it in' – at an early stage. This incident jumped into a higher stage quickly with no apparent warning. After the incident Trevor spent time on his own in his room and I was comforted by Stuart and then debriefed by my Head of Home. When Trevor stays in his room or goes back to his seat it is a good sign. If he is in/out of his room hovering I know to be careful. After a while you can read his body language although it is not always clear why he is agitated.

About two hours later I sat next to Trevor in his favourite chair. Trevor kept looking down but was quiet and calm. He tapped his hand on mine and I responded. He then tapped me further up the arm and I copied. I then felt able to look at him and say something like 'Everything OK, now Trevor?' The tap game is a good sign!

The thing that came home to me after the incident was how important communication really is. He had recently moved from one residential home to this one. Trevor probably did not fully understand what I said about going to put the switch on in the office and he must have thought that I was not going to put the TV on for him. This must have made him feel very confused or anxious. Additionally, one of his favourite members of staff due in at 8 a.m. could not get in to work and he may have been missed. Trevor has no verbal communication and he does not use sign or rebus symbols. Trevor appears to understand much of what staff say to him providing it is simple and clear, but he relies greatly on routines and the environment.

Commentary on case study 4 – Martin Bertulis

This case is one where things happened really quickly and the member of staff had to be more reactive and had to defend herself until help arrived. This is a real situation which can occur in any setting. I would like to think that training directly helped here to make Carol safe. It may be that autopilot took over for part of the time. However even when 'autopilot' was employed the correct ethos and underlying values were still in evidence.

The calm markers in the bedroom and in his favourite chair are clear to see. Some kind of repair process is also extremely important for both staff and student when there has been a flare-up like this.

Case study 5 – Steve McGreevy (RSW 2)

I have had to look back several months to find an incident which involved a difficult confrontation between myself and Trevor. I will try to describe the circumstances as best I can.

It involved me making a request/demand of Trevor that he had a bath. I had been working with him for a couple of months and felt reasonably confident in pursuing the issue with him, although he clearly did not want to have a bath and was aware he had not bathed for a couple of days. I recall that I had mentioned the idea several times in a casual manner but was getting no response. I also asked other staff on shift to 'jolly him along'! As the evening drew on I decided I needed to be more insistent. It was my belief that Trevor responded well to staff who 'stood their ground' and I felt I could do this without giving Trevor the impression I was aggressively dictating to him. However Trevor responded by pushing me across a room. I resisted this and Trevor scratched the back of both my hands. Trevor then ran to his room.

As the incident occurred several months ago, it is difficult to recall the emotional responses I felt at the time. I remember questioning my actions preceding Trevor's aggressive behaviour and feeling very hurt that Trevor could behave that way towards me! I remember feeling upset and somewhat betrayed, as my intentions had been good. I was surprised at how angry I felt.

Later I was able to talk to others on the staff team and put the situation into perspective. I felt I had been right to 'stand my ground' and this would benefit my relationship with Trevor in the future, although it upset both of us at the time. Trevor calmed fairly quickly but I had painful scars on my hands for several days after the incident.

Commentary on case study 5 – Martin Bertulis

Clear antecedents to Trevor becoming anxious and angry are demands or requests being placed upon him. It is, however, not always clear what Trevor perceives as a demand. Equally there are good reasons why sometimes demands need to be made – they are part of life. Our duty of care involves ensuring each student has a bath every few days.

The member of staff talks about trying to jolly Trevor along, but eventually needing to stand his ground. A member of staff who is very good and very effective with Trevor describes this approach as 'Bossy in a nice way!' This style could be described as insisting without dictating. The voice needs to be firm and clear but in control and calm. The body needs to be firmly rooted and wide using slow clear movements. Too much hand waving is probably not helpful.

The debriefing system is briefly alluded to, where quite destructive and negative feelings can be allowed and be put in the right place to avoid damaging good practice. Debriefing is mentioned on several occasions by staff and is covered in the systems, training and support section. We tend to use two types. Firstly there is the direct aftermath session, which ideally should be almost immediately after the incident, where the member of staff is allowed to do what they need to do (within reason) to leave the feelings at work. There is discussion as to whether this session needs to be with a senior member of staff or a colleague – there are arguments for both approaches. Staff often feel more able to open up to their direct peers and be very angry, upset and generally 'out of order'. Sometimes several members of staff in the same house or class have been involved, and here it may be better to have an outside debriefing to stop the difficult feelings circulating around the house group. In many ways it is most important that the session takes place relatively quickly.

A later second debriefing session should happen later on for analysing and learning from the incident. I have found that advising people on alternative approaches to the incident 10 minutes after it has finished can provoke a further incident with the member of staff!

Concluding thoughts – Martin Bertulis

In this concluding section I will discuss several aspects of the service and staff perspectives which initially seem quite disparate. However it is clear that there are direct links.

31

As an employer MacIntyre Care and Womaston School needs to find ways of helping staff to work humanely and professionally with behaviours which naturally evoke quite primitive responses. We have to ensure good teamwork and an understanding of the policies and ethos of the school – the words 'passion' and 'ownership' come to mind. If you have these you'll be able to develop your skills and succeed, without them, learned skills are not enough.

From an individual staff perspective it is interesting and amazing to see how often members of staff bounce back from assaults and intrusions which could so easily diminish and destroy their self-esteem. Why do they keep coming back? Having spoken to members of staff involved in the five case studies, there are recurring and unifying themes. Everybody talked about teamwork and a sense of belonging to a group who share the desire to help students to make real changes, albeit small ones at times. It was clear that staff found the work 'interesting' or 'not boring'. A recurring theme was that staff relish the challenge of trying to understand a person's world, to see why some things work and others fail, and why the same approach can have differing results. Additionally many staff talk about facing their own fears and a pride in coming back to the job even in adversity.

A common thread which pervaded the discussions was that if the level of violence, both potential and actual, goes past a certain level then it is possible to lose sight of the rewards of the job – fear and depression can easily set in. I think that the balanced view that experiencing violence is part of the job, but that it doesn't happen all the time is common in a healthy individual in a healthy team.

So how do we create and maintain the ethos of positivity and ownership of the task? In my view the culture is set and supported by the ethos of the central organisation which encourages service users and students to expect respect and understanding by building services which aim to be needs led. There is a culture of positive, value-based training using a variety of approaches including Gentle Teaching, Intensive Interaction and Rational Emotive Therapy. This eclectic approach gives staff a variety of skills to use in different settings and with different individuals. The policy for dealing with violence is a weighty document currently under review, which informs much of the work of Womaston School emphasising appropriate staff support and training. The document focuses on violence but the approaches and systems set out apply equally well to other types of challenging behaviour.

At a school, house and class level we aim to develop a culture of enquiry. This helps to separate the behaviour from the person and listen to the behaviour. Seeing behaviour as communication, i.e. something to be understood, helps to 'unload' behaviour from excessive moral judgement. Clearly there is a place for learning to behave appropriately in a variety of settings, but right–wrong arguments can be unhelpful or damaging and may create thoughts and feelings about revenge and punishment rather than support and understanding.

This term 'culture of enquiry' and how it is achieved needs further discussion. The school has many regular meetings and training sessions. Clearly meetings need to have a specific purpose but they can also have secondary spin-offs. The house and education meetings look at the nuts and bolts issues as well as deeper issues about how what we do may be perceived by the students.

Practice supervisions are now more commonplace (although not yet with every member of staff). Here staff are able to reflect on both staff and student behaviour and what it may mean. An understanding of human emotional development and group processes is developed alongside behavioural techniques and theories. Knowledge and processes from these sessions help to inform the more direct planning meetings about students, i.e. the core group meeting.

A crucial and simple tenet we hold is that if staff are supported and 'looked after' (not patronised) then they can make a better job of supporting students. The system of individual and group support and supervision pervades the entire staff team. The school is split into smaller teams which may help each other out in a crisis, i.e. when the dreaded lergy strikes! However, the development of membership of the small team which is part of the larger team is absolutely essential in supporting good practice. There is real ownership of the task, and this ownership involves administration, domestic and support staff. Training in education care teams is proving useful in developing 24-hour thinking.

It may be useful to point out that much of the success achieved with individuals like Trevor comes from previous knowledge and success. Success really does breed success, although at times it feels like one step forward, two steps back.

Detailed records of progress are kept, which help us not only modify what we do but also aid us in seeing small progress which would not be easily noticed on a day-to-day basis. I am aware of some scepticism about why we record things, who it is for and, whether it is helpful. I have heard it said that we can never truly record what is going on, thus records could distort our view of a person. Apart from the issues of accountability to the student, parents and service purchasers, a sensible mixture of quantitative and qualitative recording is essential adequately to listen to and understand behaviour.

Finally, are we helping Trevor with all of our meetings, training and theory? He still gets anxious at times and I suspect he will for a long time to come. Since he has come to us he has developed a wider and more interesting community presence. He knows and can work with more people. He continues to learn to cope with changes with relatively limited verbal skills, and of course we know him better now and really like him.

References

McGee, J. J., Menolascino, F. J., Hobbs, D. C., Menousek, P. E. (1987) *Gentle Teaching: A Nonaversive Approach for Helping Persons with Mental Retardation.* New York: Human Science Press.

Nind, M. and Hewett, D. (1994) *Access to Communication: Developing the Basics of Communication with People with Severe Learning Difficulties Through Intensive Interaction.* London: David Fulton Publishers.

Chapter 3

A flat for one – social service provision at the extreme

Nicki Bond and Don O'Connor

Flat 7: how the project started – Nicki and Don

Some people with learning disabilities just find it too difficult to live with other people. We like them to live in groups, it is easier for us, but in the end Andrew's difficulties with other residents, and the difficulties his behaviour made for them, meant that he received, for a while, an increasingly personally tailored service. Living with other people with learning disabilities is only half the problem, however. Even with what was ultimately a provision designed to his needs and behaviour, he still had the difficulty of living with the staff.

Andrew is 37 years old, he is a large man, six feet tall and weighing approximately 16 stones. He has receding brown hair and green eyes. He was born after a late toxaemia pregnancy ending in induced labour. He suffered early seizures and was diagnosed as having epilepsy. At seven years he was diagnosed as having a learning disability and autism.

He attended a school for children with learning disabilities until he was 18 and then he lived with his mother, father and sister. He also had a very close relationship with his grandparents, particularly his grandfather, who was a retired charge nurse and spent a great deal of time with Andrew throughout his childhood and teenage years. His grandparents lived very close to him and apparently Andrew's grandfather did some sort of activity with Andrew every day, either walking or going to the playground or visiting friends of his where he used to work. Andrew's grandparents died and he misses them very much.

After leaving school Andrew went to live at a large hospital run by a voluntary organisation. This was expected to be a permanent placement but Andrew was refused re-admission after a weekend visit home. Andrew had lived there for five years and, as Tommy Cooper would say, 'just like that', he never returned. He was never given an opportunity to say goodbye to anyone. Andrew still becomes distressed if he hears any mention of that hospital. The reasons for this distress were never explored (his mother felt it unwise). His mother has told me that a fellow resident was given the responsibility of 'minding' Andrew. But she remembers Andrew walking home alone once (several miles); the walks with his grandad certainly came in useful. This caused a great deal of anxiety for Andrew's mother as, when she returned to the hospital with him several hours later, she found he hadn't been missed. So, he returned to live with his parents again.

He was admitted to a large day centre, which he attended from 1983 to 1993. His attendance was good – he went Monday to Friday to the special needs unit. Over about one to two years Andrew's behaviour was causing some concern. After an application for additional funding, Andrew was allocated his own 1:1 worker. An arrangement was made for Andrew to move out of the special needs unit and into the main centre. This move was seen as a positive one for Andrew, and all went well for approximately five months when, again, Andrew's behaviour was a cause for concern.

It was arranged for him to attend a day centre (2) for people who challenge for one week's assessment and return to the other day centre (1) the following week. However, Andrew's mother strongly objected to him returning to day centre 1 and he remained at day centre 2. He did not get an opportunity to say his goodbyes and again left in a negative way. He reacts very negatively to any mention of the day centre 1, just as he did to mention of the hospital he lived at.

In fact, I remember an incident about two years ago when I (Don) had borrowed the centre's minibus for a drive out in the country with Andrew. I had already parked the minibus in our car park. On returning from the drive I decided rather than all of us get out and then me returning the bus next door I would park the bus outside the day centre first and we could then all walk back together. It was a bad decision, as I had barely got the bus in the gates when Andrew started screaming inconsolably. You have never seen anyone reverse a minibus as quickly as I did that day!

The behaviours recorded at day centre 1 ranged from self-injurious behaviour such as nail biting and finger sucking (to the point of making his fingers bleed), scratching, pinching his arms, attacking staff and clients, attempting to get people on the floor, screaming and crying. It was also recorded that Andrew had been experiencing difficulty with his sexuality which would sometimes result in him attaching himself to female members of staff in the emotional sense or lunging at them. Andrew's mother was apparently experiencing no problems at home with Andrew at this time.

Andrew remained at day centre 2 for about a year before being asked to leave as a result of his challenge to the service they could offer him. The incidents of aggression were similar to those at the previous day centre. Andrew's mother reported at this time that Andrew was coming home in a 'bad mood' and shouting and scratching her.

Andrew was also receiving some respite care at Flat 7, where he now lives, and there was growing concern then at the increase in Andrew's challenging behaviour and aggressive outbursts. The proposed plan at the time was for Andrew to move into Flat 7, despite growing concerns regarding Andrew's tolerance of the female resident he would share with.

A period of assessment at Gallipolli House, a residential facility specialising in working with people with challenging behaviours was decided upon. They would look particularly at the question of the suitability of Flat 7 for Andrew in the light of the increased tension between himself and the client he would be living with that was arising during his respite stays. Andrew actually lived at Gallipoli House for one year before moving to Flat 7 on Valentine's Day 1995.

Establishing Flat 7 – Nicki

Due to difficult placements and the parents' inability to cope any more, a section of Hazelmere House was set up as a specialist unit to accommodate people with very challenging behaviours. Hazelmere is basically a large old-style 1970s hostel, though in recent years it has been modernised and divided up into flats with their own kitchens. A new flat had been built as Flat 7 and Andrew and Betty had in fact moved in and been there for two weeks before I arrived as team leader. For all sorts of reasons the project was set up very hurriedly in the end, and I couldn't get released from my previous job in time to be in post at the start.

I started working with children in a children's home in Sussex. I was very attracted to working with children with challenging behaviour and always seemed to be given the challenging kids to work with. I then moved into working with young adults with autism, and I worked with them for about four years. I gained more senior positions as I went along. I started working for Hertfordshire Social Services at another residential establishment, but I was very unhappy there and wanted to be transferred. When the job in Flat 7 came up, I thought 'This sounds like me', so I applied for it and got it.

The staffing of the flat was worked out quite hurriedly as well, though we were fortunate with a few of the personalities. There was no day-care provision or activities arranged for Andrew – we were doing that from scratch too. Actually there still are no other day-care activities; it remains one of the working principles with Andrew that the staff who work with him residentially also facilitate the day activities. This has gradually developed over the time of the project and works well now. Betty was attending out-of-house day activities and some staff already knew her, so that was not so much of a difficulty. However, for Andrew the first weeks were about confusion and a lack of structure. We struggled just to manage and contain him and get to know him. There was quite a bit of understandable fear among the team and we were taking injuries. We took a hard look at some of the management strategies that we had inherited, dropped the ones that were getting us into trouble and more or less started again from scratch.

It was definably the worst possible start for the project, but ultimately I think it perversely worked in our favour. We had no choice but to buckle down and work at sorting things out, get to know Andrew, sort out procedures and structures, have some staff reshuffling, learn how to work and survive together. I think the staff have maintained a very flexible attitude since that time.

I remember that we had to work on our expectations. There were all these expectations that we were there to cure Andrew. This was an expensive resource in terms of staffing, I think social services naturally expects some kind of 'cure' outcome from that sort of outlay, but probably we expected that from ourselves as well. Gradually, our expectation changed to surviving effectively and living with Andrew in some sort of harmony. Of course, having got our expectations realistic and settled, working forward with Andrew became more possible. I think there was general surprise when Don suggested earlier this year that the time was right for another resident to move into the flat with Andrew.

- confusion and lack of understanding about what is happening around him – autism

- learning disabilities – unknown origin

- still at early stage of emotional development

- anxiety as a virtually permanent mood

- very negative about himself – lack of self-esteem

- difficulty forming attachments and having relationships he can understand

- epilepsy – tonic clinic – mostly well controlled

- at stressful times – epileptic seixures and a long build-up phase

- ankle injury re-occurrence occasionally

- behaviour can be triggered by pain

- history of behaviour difficulties all his life – these behaviours were part of his lifestyle

- very high general arousal levels

- bereavement

- losses in his life – not having the chance to say goodbye. Moves – too many in too short a time

---

Figure 3.1 Things we think contribute to Andrew's challenging behaviours

First steps – Nicki

The team had conflicts in the early stages as to the best tactics with Andrew. There were seven staff appointed on a full-time basis and we had to learn the hard way to sit and talk and find resolutions to our differences. The hardest things were deciding on the right approaches and then getting consistency across the team. The staff team fluctuated in terms of membership for a long time, but then we had two male staff join us as agency workers, and they remained with us for a long time on that basis, becoming good team members. One of the advantages perhaps was that being agency staff, they were happy to be told how to work and they fitted in well with the style we started to develop.

We identified early on that Andrew and Betty were not compatible in their needs and that it was difficult to contain Andrew's aggressive behaviour as he was being challenged on an hourly basis by Betty being verbally abusive to him and triggering him. We were then becoming involved in restraint situations to protect Betty and separate Andrew from her. It was often difficult to maintain her safety – we couldn't always get her out of the way because she refused to move.

This was a very tough time. The staff had various years of experience or very little at all. The biggest hurdle to overcome was achieving consistency with attitudes towards the clients and attitudes towards approaches to take. A popular one within the unit at the time was that the hands-on approach towards behaviours exhibited and punitive atmosphere was the right thing. The thought of leaving the vicinity to allow the client some space to calm down was greeted by sheer horror by some of the staff. It meant we weren't doing our job properly and it showed we were backing down or scared of the client! Too right, I was, when you're greeted by a 16 stone man who has entered his 'crisis' point and was attempting to rip my clothes off – scared is one way of putting it!

Trying to make this situation better was, of course, my responsibility and I had to go through my own learning process. I felt the weight of everyone looking to me to lead and at times I really didn't know the best way forward. I believed deep down that we should not have been restraining him and it was not doing anybody any good – certainly not him. Every time we restrained him he became more aggressive, biting people, but we always felt forced to restrain him. On the one hand some of us were saying there are other ways we know we would like to work with Andrew, but we were contradicting ourselves by restraining him frequently because we didn't have the choice.

However, once we started implementing techniques to help overcome behaviour and proved (for want of a better word) that they were more productive and positive, people did begin to agree and become more confident about approaches they were using.

The problem is, as soon as a client is labelled with challenging behaviour sometimes that is all that is seen. I remember the community nurse observing Andrew in the unit one day when he was very partial to scratching other people's hands when distressed. He became very agitated and upset and everyone (staff) in the unit stood very still waiting to see what was going to happen. However, this time my gut reaction was to approach him and offer tenderness and my hands to hold. I could feel the pure tension in the air and people's minds whirring with thoughts like, 'She's told us to back away and here she is approaching him and giving him her hands!' Luck was on my side, he responded really well and had a good cry and held my hands pleasantly throughout. He calmed and went back to drawing.

All the staff and the community nurse who had observed this were full of questions about why I had used this approach and not the agreed backing away one. My only conclusion then and now is that Andrew is a person first and at times we all need reassurance and human contact, not the opposite. I had read that situation well and made the right judgement I think, but, explaining to other staff how I did it was difficult.

I also hope that this incident was part of the process which enabled staff to see that with all the training and professional qualifications we have, that the most fundamental approach to keep in mind in our work is that these are human beings, people with feelings, desires and needs that are as individual as anybody else and deserve to be treated as such.

Joining the staff of Flat 7 – Don

After I left school, I was a cobbler for two and a half years in Mallow, County Cork. I came to England in 1988 and worked at Fairfield Hospital, a large psychiatric hospital, as a nursing assistant. I had a good deal of varied experience there – working with the elderly and in the secure ward for over a year – which was horrible. I worked in a flat with people with challenging behaviour for one and a half years, then to a purpose built flat, bigger than Flat 7, again for people with challenging behaviour. I enjoyed that, for one and a half years with two clients who were very physically aggressive. I had a few other experiences in residential work with people with learning disabilities. One was in a situation where the residents were so quiet and well-behaved that I moved on because I found it boring. I heard about the vacancy here and thought that it probably wouldn't be boring. I was right.

I first met Andrew when I came to work in Flat 7 in April 1995. Andrew was very curious of this stranger who skulked around in the background, but after an introduction and an explanation of who I was and why I was there, he knew who I was – that I was just another member of staff. This type of introduction was probably one of the many that Andrew has had over the years.

Andrew was providing the staff in place with some very interesting challenging incidents. They all dealt with the incidents in different ways initially, probably due to the different skill mix within the team. Andrew also tended to 'focus' most of his aggression and anxieties onto one particular member of staff. The staff member could differ from week to week or month to month.

Andrew's anxieties were mostly based around two things. He showed continuous anxiety about what was happening during each day, the ordering of normal routines, who was on duty, when were we going out. There were also the 'events' that happened in his life. Some examples of these events are the Easter holiday, Whitsun, Andrew's birthday and Christmas.

He would seek reassurance that these events were happening by saying 'Easter holiday' in a very demanding tone. He generally picked one member of staff, approached them and shouted the words 'Easter holidays'. The staff member had to reassure Andrew that Easter was in March – two Sundays, he would be visiting his parents on Easter Saturday, his Dad would pick up him, etc. This process often took five to ten minutes as Andrew would constantly repeat the word over and over and the member of staff had to do the same. In the early stages of knowing Andrew these incidents mostly led to Andrew attacking the staff member, being physically restrained, although occasionally he accepted the staff member's response and sat down. These incidents could happen up to ten times a day, and as soon as Easter was over he would start to seek reassurance about the next important event in his life.

As these incidents were very 'tense' for both the staff member and Andrew, the outcome (in my opinion) often depended on how reassured Andrew felt by the staff member who was 'dealing with the incident'. He seemed to sense any signs of nerves or insecurities that members of staff had, and generally they would be the staff members that he would mostly focus his attentions on. He would often be happy/calm for a morning shift but as soon as he saw a certain member of staff he would become anxious and would start talking about these events.

One thing that didn't help was that Betty was around many times when Andrew was talking about these events – she would often say to him 'You're not going home for Easter. Why don't you just shut up!'

When Andrew first lived in Flat 7 he had very little structure to his day. He didn't have any day-care placement (and still doesn't) and spent most of his day doing puzzles, building bricks, having stories read to him or colouring. Colouring was his favourite activity and he often got through a hundred sheets of paper in a shift. I often wonder how many sheets of paper he has coloured in his life. He would colour in quick left to right strokes with one colour until the page was full and then choose another colour and go over the first colour (making very pretty pictures). He liked the colours he was creating. It also had a calming effect on him, probably due to the rhythm he had going.

Andrew's only routine when he came to live in Flat 7 was visiting his parents house for the weekend every fortnight and going for a drive with his Dad on the Saturday he wasn't at his parents. These two things caused Andrew great anxiety, again seeking lots of reassurance they would be happening. Dealing with these anxieties often led to aggressive outbursts from Andrew.

For me, depending on who I was working with, I could feel comfortable dealing with the incidents or often very uncomfortable. It depended on whether I was feeling other staff were vulnerable or I was vulnerable. Different staff often dealt with incidents differently, and the ones who were anxious or fussy themselves were likely to be the main focus of Andrew's negative attention and were almost sure to meet with 'confrontation'.

During a time of high anxiety it was very difficult to put any distance between yourself and Andrew if he was focusing his anxiety onto you in particular. He would stand very close to you and, as he is 6 feet tall, he mostly looks down on people. If the incident led to aggression a second member of staff would intervene and hold Andrew's arm as he would be trying to scratch the staff member. He would then be encouraged to go to his bedroom to calm down while the members of staff held his arms. We learned in time to change this approach as Andrew began to bite people who were holding him and two members of staff were badly injured.

At the time we were closely monitoring Andrew's behaviour and looking out for triggers to try and avoid these confrontational episodes. This learning process for us was very intense, and slowly improved over time, but unfortunately due to the stress, violence, pressure and other factors in the first 12 months Andrew lived in Flat 7, various staff left or chose to work in a different flat. This added to Andrew's anxiety as he found strangers difficult and we had to employ a lot of agency staff. I remember this being a time of great frustration as I felt the regular staff were making progress with Andrew, but we were often hindered by the lack of consistency caused by using many agency staff. There was certainly a fear factor around working with Andrew. Some of the agency staff's attitude and ethos were very different to ours. We learnt to have available a co-ordination sheet. This was a two-side briefing sheet to explain to agency staff at the beginning of a shift what we did, why, and how we did it, particularly non-confrontation, using space, defusing. This was mostly really helpful, but not all of the temps could learn quickly in one shift, then we wouldn't see them again, it would be someone else.

Often we were doing everything in shift and telling some staff to just stay out of the way as much as possible or generally protecting them. It would be very easy for someone that had never met Andrew to say one wrong word and trigger his anxiety. It felt like there was so much information to tell new agency staff. In fact the information we passed on to people about the type of incident which may occur, how Andrew would more than likely focus his attention on them, etc., would often freak people out. It wasn't uncommon for someone to change their mind at the start of the shift and not work in our flat, or if they did they often refused to return. It was hard to blame them as really they must have felt like lambs to the slaughter.

We were also lucky to have some very good long-term agency workers who Andrew seemed to accept after an initial testing period. Incidents were still occurring but were being dealt with more consistently. Two or three agency workers practically worked full time and for me it was really the first time it felt like there was any real stability in the team and we were all working along the same lines. Communication was essential between staff and I often felt it was unfortunate that agency staff were excluded from things like training or even attending weekly staff meetings. By this time Nicki had got good working structures organised and she was strict about staff doing recordings, reading briefing sheets, following agreed styles and procedures, staying on the ball.

Bad work, mishaps, accidents, wrong turnings, staff morale – Nicki

In the beginning, before I started at the unit, Andrew moved in with almost no accompanying information or life history. Staff were left with a blank sheet, no training, no experience, but lots of behaviours occurring every day.

The approach was three staff on shift with the two clients, men only dealing with the incidents and they would physically remove Andrew to another 'time out' room. Great, especially as you had to go through at least two doors to get there – three men, two doors and lots of behaviours – not a good mix.

We learnt to relax some of our early attitudes. Betty seemed obsessed over a particular personal item. This needed washing every morning and the old 'common' approach was not to give it back to her until late in the day. Once we began returning it as soon as it was washed, she was much happier and relaxed instead of tense, aggressive and tearful. This also benefited Andrew of course. It was not much effort to get it done as quickly as possible, but we had to overcome some attitudes around 'she'll get it back when we can do it, not the moment she wants it.'.

We had a discussion as a team as to how to deal with Andrew's self-injurious behaviour. He particularly bit his fingers so badly that he would have numerous infections and very sore fingers. Our initial line was to hold his hands and arms to try and calm him down. Big mistake. He bit a staff member instead. After such incidents, we decided on a completely different approach. We offered reassurance and support while he was doing it, but did not try and stop him. We learnt very quickly that as soon as you use a hands-on approach in any situation it can just makes things worse. This focused us very well on learning how to defuse him, particularly with use of our voices.

Morale became very low when Betty was moved out of the unit. The decision was ultimately taken because we just could not guarantee her physical well-being, even staffed as we were. There surely must also be some questions about two people who really didn't seem to like each other being required to live together in the same flat, just because they both have challenging behaviours. Whatever the rationale, we could not help feeling that we were failures, that we had done a bad job by not keeping her safe. Some staff felt unsupported and two people left the unit. That left us with even more inconsistency and once again we had agency staff that hadn't been to us previously. At this time our practices were obviously being looked at and questioned, but luckily we came through that alright.

Andrew's behaviour did improve once Betty was moved out. One of his main triggers had been taken away and staff could at least remove themselves from the situation if he became agitated because they didn't have to worry about Betty. However, as a team, we were still caring for Betty, albeit in an adjacent flat. Trying now to run two separate units effectively was very difficult, but we did manage. When we had three staff on duty in Andrew's flat, and one of them was a weak link or somebody Andrew was currently focusing on, we could select that person to be working with Betty.

Around this time we had a new member of staff join who was particularly strong and we had some more training given which did pick up the staff's morale. We also continued to change our approach to Andrew so that hands-on contact was avoided.

Moving on – Nicki and Don

The greatest developments then started occurring. We were getting better and better at tuning-in to and recognising how Andrew needed an effective day to be organised and structured and we were becoming more consistent and effective with the challenging incidents. Andrew likes having a very simple, predictable, structure to what is going to happen and when it will happen. We learnt to go with this, get things like that right for him and to acknowledge that there weren't any details that were too basic to be attended to.

For example, Coronation Street was on at a regular time, every night and he could visibly see on the screen when it was finished. After Coronation Street he would have a foot spa, after the foot spa at 9.00 p.m. he had some supper, and after supper he would go and get changed, come back out and have another cup of tea, then go to his room. Simple things, but then if there were any long gaps you could read him a story and just bridge those gaps. So to him his evening was quite full, predictable and relaxed – very reassuring for him.

These routines were expanded because they worked so well. Mornings became like that too. We could fill his day with things which we would put in his dairy in words and pictures which we could reassure him with regularly. He had his own diary and we would write down the events of each day, tightly described. So any time he started getting agitated you could take the edge off the agitation, you could say, 'Hey Andrew, say come and sit down next to me and we'll go through your diary'. So then he wasn't leaning over you and in your face, you were sitting together and the member of staff was gently going through everything which would be happening that day.

We tried to structure the whole week with the same predictability, introduce things that would happen on the same day, like swimming and hydrotherapy and make the week similarly predictable and reassuring.

Building a relationship

The really important thing about the times spent sitting drawing with Andrew or going through his diary over and over again, or reading him a story was that these activities helped staff to build up a relationship. It meant that staff could then approach, 'Right, okay Andrew, shall we do some colouring or shall we read a story?'

Because we started paying a lot of attention to the minute detail of a very basic structure of events throughout each and every day, we increasingly had many, perhaps minor interactions with Andrew, based on stuff he was vitally interested in. These engagements were also effective for him because they supplied him with information he wanted and he was therefore having these numerous but brief and meaningful interactions which were interesting for him because they were about his concerns.

This was happening at the most basic of levels but at one that was right for Andrew. One of the things we realised quite early on was that the more you focused on Andrew, the more stressed out he became because he could not cope with all that attention. So it needed to be quite positive and focused attention on his terms.

We were getting him to take more control of his life. He became more confident to do things like come and ask us for a cup of tea rather than us ask him regularly if he wanted it. He would come and say, 'tea', whereas before he would wait to be given one – he had more control and again it was relationship building on a basic level. This seems like a small advance, but for us it felt fundamental and a real milestone. Because he at last had a situation where staff could focus just on his lifestyle needs, uncompromised, he was starting to get his environment right and we were learning how to relate to him properly. For him, the people around him were becoming more and more consistent in the way that they related to him, more tuned-in to the potential difficulties he had with normal daily events.

Consistent approach

Also, we dealt with his aggressive behaviour better after Betty left. We didn't have to use a hands-on approach so much. This was vitally important because that was a big change to the past way of dealing with things. Andrew was still lunging at us but suddenly, instead of restraining him, we had the option of avoiding him. The flat is quite well designed – the living room has a 1970s style slatted partition which is quite easy to duck behind. From there you can still talk to him and make eye contact, but having removed yourself from his immediate presence. Slightly strange perhaps, but an effective ploy.

We all had agreed by then that we would use a consistent approach to Andrew's build-up. The tactic of removing him to his room became more and more effective. We would ask him to go to his room when he was becoming agitated. Sometimes we would walk him there, not restraining or forcing him, but perhaps gently holding an arm, one person on either side and prompting. We did this consistently, and he started to go simply when we asked him. We felt that he started to like it, to be on his own and calm down. Sometimes, particularly in the early stages, he would shred his clothes while he was in there, but that was okay, it's much better than shredding people. We told him that. We encouraged it, rather than saying 'Don't do that! That's bad!'. In time, it got to the point where he would take himself away without being asked. One of us would say, 'Where's Andrew?' Someone else would say, 'Oh he was getting worked up and he went off to his room'. He started to learn that he had available alternatives to violence. He could sit with us and go through his diary, relate and communicate, he could go to his room and be alone to calm down.

Our style at times of crisis became more of a style which we were all using. All the team learnt to use their voices when Andrew was 'high', to speak slowly and reassuringly. Members of the team were openly evaluating things like use of eye contact and how close to get at certain times. We had a repertoire of defusers we all used: the diary, his room, a sit down with someone on the sofa for a chat. Everyone became more positive and didn't mind repeating themselves to be reassuring. Staff were less 'controlling' with their voices and the way they approached Andrew, but we were controlling him much better.

Record keeping and monitoring behaviours – Nicki

We developed our documentation to the point where our routines were focused around the use of four sheets:

1. positive evaluation forms (see Figure 3.2);
2. incident records;
3. ABC charts;
4. specific behaviour tick charts.

Sheet 1 was extremely useful as the wording on them made staff record the actual incident and then look at what good work was carried out during the incident. Doing the recordings on this sheet really contributed to our management and teamwork. There would usually be at least two of us filling a sheet in and the discussion which went with it became interesting and enjoyable. Sheets 2 and 3 helped us to work on looking at Andrew's trigger points and becoming more aware and familiar with what were 'hotspots' in the day, together with the appreciation that his behaviour usually didn't just happen without an environmental cause or something 'inside' Andrew, his thoughts and anxieties – or both.

Sheet 4 was very factual, giving an easy way of recording the numbers of the type of incidents that usually occurred. It gave us a clear way to look for any patterns of behaviour emerging and for transferring data for analysis.

At a later stage all the information gathered on sheet 4 was collated and put on to a graph to identify the following things:

- the increase/decrease of violent incidents;
- the increase/decrease of self-injurious behaviour;
- the amount of incidents occurring with each staff member.

This last point was extremely important as sometimes staff were focused on in a negative way by Andrew and it gave us an opportunity to examine what might be happening to evoke reactions from him. It also identified in a very factual sense if there were any members of staff having significantly more incidents than others. We could then think about ways to help remedy this. This wasn't particularly welcomed by the staff who were having difficulties but increasingly we all accepted the necessity.

Date: Time: Place: Staff making evaluation:

Description of incident: what took place and if possible, why (think about factors and triggers perhaps):

What procedure(s) was used to manage the incident?:

What did staff do that was good work and/or effective? (List examples of this even if the incident ultimately became unmanageable):

Thoughts for the future:

Figure 3.2 Positive evaluation sheet

Of course, we were able to have proper time available to carry out recordings, but having had this experience of doing it so thoroughly, we both feel that the need to do good documentation, no matter what, will always be with us. The recordings and discussions also provided us with training for the future and the evaluation of good working methods among the team. As the manager of the unit it also assisted me in identifying skills used by staff that were not always evident to me if I wasn't on shift and gave me the chance to feed back on good ideas.

Training, talking, developing team practices – Nicki

We did a lot of work on our attitudes, individually and as a team. Talking about them became a theme, not always an easy one. This developed mainly because in the early days some of the ways of thinking about Andrew's behaviour were negative. Some people could not get beyond the thinking that Andrew's behaviour was premeditated, that he knew what he was doing and was aiming to hurt people. This was evident in the comments made, for example: 'He did it on purpose – he waited for me to leave before he got up and did it' (ABC sheet). Although this particular comment was true, the interpretation of his actions was personal and wrongly interpreted and likely to result in negative attitudes where we just blamed Andrew all the time. Even though Andrew did think about it, did it on purpose and waited for his moment, we can't hold him solely responsible for being difficult and then have a negative general attitude toward him. That doesn't get us anywhere, and being very negative to Andrew didn't help him to stop doing it. He had already had years of that and he was still doing these things.

We had some team training on challenging behaviours, which was really useful and contributed to this main staff development we learnt to do – we talked all the time. There was a significant training day we had together in the late summer of 1995 when we brainstormed lists of what we knew about our work with Andrew. These were:

- things we knew about Andrew;
- what Andrew likes;
- Andrew's challenges;
- autism;
- things we have done well;
- strategies;
- communication;
- how to offer reassurance and security;
- incident management, warning signs, breakaways.

This was, for us, a brilliant day. To be able to sit together and summarise all the various aspects of Andrew's behaviour and look at the trigger points for incidents, but also look at what sort of person Andrew was, what his likes were and what his personality was like. I feel it really got us in touch with him as a person and not just someone who exhibited negative behaviours.

It also enabled us to build on the positives about ourselves. We worked hard to get a good picture of how well we were doing rather than simply focusing on our shortcomings. We acknowledged the growth in our approach to Andrew, particularly the increasing effectiveness of our incident management and the setting of predictable routines. We wrote all of this down together that day, doing some good, straight talking with each other of course, but listing on big sheets of paper all of the positives in our work.

We were benefiting from having some good time during shifts to do our talking and evaluation. If Andrew was in a good mood, he would often prefer to sit alone occupying himself, with no-one else too near. This would give us frequent episodes of 15 minutes or so when the staff on shift were able to sit and write records and evaluations, talk and think about practice – out of Andrew's earshot of course. As our morale and attitudes improved, we became quite well focused on the need to do this, and the whole team became good at not talking to each other about what was on television last night, but on getting better at our work with Andrew. We do recognise that the set-up of our unit allowed us this 'luxury'. We have worked in other situations where time for this has to be found somehow.

Recording and evaluating got us into good habits of positive discussion which focused our teamwork. It's often not easy to do good documentation, but we were enjoying it most of the time. It was so vitally important to us to have the statistical records which told us whether Andrew was having more or fewer difficult incidents.

To the present day – Don

Nicki got pregnant, which was actually really good (she thought so too) because it gave her a lot more time out of direct contact, although she did still get involved quite a lot. However, for reasons of her own safety she was spending less time on direct contact and more on supervising, writing working guidelines and observations about Andrew. She also prepared for leaving by really detailing and writing down the framework of our work with Andrew. She left at Christmas 1995 and I took over as team leader.

By that time we had in place all of the basics of the approach to Andrew, which still pretty much follow the same pattern now, though of course they continue to develop and grow: the foot spas, Coronation Street, the swimming, all the little routines through the day which we have developed to help some of Andrew's more major anxieties. We've continued to work on our relationships with him and our ability to manage the difficult moments, and I think he gets a great deal of security from the consistency of the staff behaviour. This aspect of structure is always there. I put a lot of time in sitting with Andrew and doing puzzles and drawings, or just talking. I remember how anxious we were at the beginning about how to start interacting with him in a way that worked, and now it has got to the stage where I'm continually relaxed when I'm working with him.

I went swimming with him for the first time in a long time last week. I was swimming with one arm and with the other I grabbed his leg. He was floating and I was spinning him around. This was something I would not have dreamed of attempting some time ago, but he was relaxed and laughing, really enjoying it.

There haven't been any serious incidents over the last 12 months. Mostly Andrew is not in the state where he will be seriously challenging or the incidents have been well defused before he's got to that point. He's still doing well with his own coping procedures, taking himself off to his room now and again. Then you stick your head round his door and say, 'How are you feeling now Andrew?'

Andrew lived on his own for a year, which gave us time to build relationships with him, create a good lifestyle, establish security and help him to be more calm generally. Last winter I was asked to meet this chap in Suffolk with a reputation for challenging behaviour – to give advice based on our experiences. Graham is from Hertfordshire and his family wanted him to move back to somewhere locally. There was a deadline for his move so some quick action was taken on making provision for him. This meant that Hazelmere had to re-organise to provide a bedsit-type accommodation with two members of staff continuously working with Graham. I worked with Graham often during that time and I started thinking that he probably wouldn't challenge Andrew in the way that Betty had. The Flat 7 team talked it over for a while. We were feeling confident about Andrew's stability and calmness. So, we started suggesting that Graham move into Flat 7 – it made sense from a staffing point of view and it was always our aim that we would work toward Andrew being able to live with others again. Andrew was fine about the suggestion when he met our prospective new resident. The situation has been working really well for the two of them for the past eight months. The only difficulty has been disagreements about the television. Graham has this little 'wind-up' where he turns off the television and waits for one of us to react. We say 'Leave the television alone please' and Andrew is happy with that, he doesn't react too negatively to Graham's provocation – he knows we will handle it I think.

At the moment the team feels good about the situation and we are looking forward positively. For a while Andrew had an expensive provision all to himself, but it seemed that this was the basic thing necessary to support him and help him get into shape to start living with other people again. Of course, it may all change at some time, Andrew may have a 'dip' or the staff group might change too much too quickly to keep up the consistency. However, we feel we have achieved some deep changes with Andrew and we've got great hopes that he will keep up his more positive ways.

Chapter 4

The challenge of Class Six

Bernard Emblem with Jill Leonard, Karen Dale,
Joanne Redmond and Ruth Bowes

An introduction to the class

This is the tale of a group of children and the adults working with them who found
themselves faced with unexpected challenges and devised novel and interesting
ways of dealing with them. It's not an account of a carefully planned programme,
it's the story of everyday but exceptional folk, whose lack of preconceived ideas,
lack of knowledge of behavioural methods, even of interactive methods *per se*,
threw them back on their natural reserves and their basic instincts, to produce an
exciting and effective way of working with young children in a special school.

Brian Frew and I once wrote of a way of working which we called activity
centred learning, or ACL. We tried to describe and systematise the good practice
we observed all around us, taking as our premise the belief that schools are
composed of groups of adults and children whose main focus is not the aims and
objectives they describe in their paperwork, but the activities they jointly engage
in (Emblem and Frew 1988).

Nind and Hewett were evolving Intensive Interaction at around the same time.
For them, the interactions between adult and child, teacher and student, or carer
and client are the main focus of interest (Nind and Hewett 1994).

Though we hadn't talked much in school about these ways of describing
teaching and learning, what evolved in Class Six can, to some extent, be
explained in terms of ACL and Intensive Interaction. The staff found themselves
focusing on the environment and the interactions within it; an emphasis on
learning rather than teaching. In the process, I watched children with limited
communication skills and challenging behaviour start to communicate more
effectively, become less disruptive, and gain access to an increasing number of
experiences and opportunities.

Millwood is a primary school for children with learning difficulties. Our story
begins at the start of a recent school year, when we found that one class of five to
seven year olds had an unusually high proportion of children with severe learning
difficulties and challenging behaviour.

We had just appointed a new teacher for the class, and we were confident that a
successful team would emerge from the partnership of two highly skilled nursery
nurses (NNEBs), and a young teacher straight from a challenging primary school
in a neighbouring authority, supported for half the week by an experienced team
leader. Jill was appointed in preference to more experienced candidates largely on
the basis of her composure, confidence and enthusiasm. They would become the

exceptional team this chapter is about. Unfortunately, Jill's LEA refused to release her in time for the beginning of the next school year – she had missed the resignation deadline by a few days. So we had to find a replacement at short notice. It wasn't a good term for us or the supply teacher, who wanted to succeed, but never managed to take control of the situation. However, this difficult term brought out new qualities and new confidence in nursery nurses Joanne and Karen, as they found themselves forced into making decisions between them about how to work with the class. It is from this inauspicious beginning that the magic which became Class Six grew. By the time Jill arrived after Christmas, she walked into an environment characterised by acceptance and respect. Fortunately, Jill, too, is a natural.

I knew something special was happening when I went to look more closely. I saw sensitivity, acceptance, an ability to spot opportunities, and to turn behaviour which I would have interpreted as challenging into opportunities for positive interactions. To observe a lesson with these three is to learn.

We hope enough of the excitement and frustration of real life remains for you to be able to believe in this as an account of on-going practice as well as a conscious attempt to relate theories about teaching and learning to a real setting.

An introduction to the approach

This year I have watched the staff in Class Six combine a position of professional detachment in which they accept, observe and hypothesise, with human involvement in which they become significant, through showing respect for the children and having something to offer them.

Accepting means accepting the person, not necessarily the behaviour. Observing leads to the formulation of hypotheses about behaviour, which will ask 'Why do they do this?' and go on to ask – 'What is it reasonable to expect of this child in this situation?' Very different behaviour is accepted from each child. This is the basis for much of the success of the class. In addition, staff implement a creative approach to more intransigent behaviour. For example:

- for David's entrenched behaviour, a more formal approach involving an individual behaviour plan was required;
- staff learned to defuse challenging situations, and to use them constructively when working with Naomi;
- when the approach was not working for John, we hypothesised that this was because he was the odd one out in the class, and moved him to a more appropriate environment.

Causes – why do they behave like this?

Much of teaching hinges on our hypotheses about why children behave as they do, since this will influence how we respond to the challenges they offer us –

effective intervention must target the right cause. When we meet children with deficits in social and communication skills, and unusual ways of behaving we must ask – are they autistic? We work on a broad definition of autism and now educate a small group of children in a discrete class using the TEACCH method (Mesibov *et al.* 1994), an approach based on the assumption that children with autism find the world chaotic and frightening, and so learn more effectively in a very predictable environment. This has been remarkably successful.

But Class Six is a group of more social children, whose behaviour seems to be largely associated with failed attempts to relate successfully. Thus, our organisation is based on theories about children's needs, based on observations of their interactions.

Children present challenging behaviour for a variety of reasons, some personal, such as difficulties with communication, some environmental, such as lack of appropriate experience. What they all have in common is that they have gained something from behaving in this way – it serves a purpose for them. They all need lots of opportunities to behave constructively and to find new ways of behaving which they (not we) find more rewarding than their previous behaviour.

The term 'challenging behaviour' was coined to put a new slant on the behaviour of children who might previously have been described as disturbed or maladjusted. It defines the behaviour, not in terms of the child, but in terms of the effect it has – this behaviour challenges other people. Our task is to decide how to respond to this challenge, in the belief that our responses can make this behaviour less likely to occur, and with a clear understanding that we can only alter children's behaviour by altering adult behaviour. According to this perspective, challenging behaviour has something to do with relationships and communications which are going wrong.

The children

Let us look at some of the 5–7 year olds in Class Six. We'll see how these ideas translate into classroom approaches, and pick up some of the themes I have used when describing adult behaviour.

I have categorised the children's needs as follows:

- children whose attempts to communicate lead to problems – Naomi, Vanessa and Carl;
- children who have very little understanding of relationships or communication – Mark;
- children who have learned to communicate and relate through aggression, disruption, or other anti-social behaviour – David, Imtiaz and John.

Children whose attempts to communicate lead to problems

These children need to develop the ability to communicate more effectively. Naomi, Vanessa and Carl all became less challenging during the year.

Naomi: 'She wants to sit on your knee'

... in which staff demonstrate acceptance and become significant by having something to offer

Naomi is desperate to communicate, or maybe just to gain attention. She does this by lots of shouting, reaching out, and eye contact. She has little more to say than 'Hiya', and wants little more than your attention, so her calls are not context sensitive – she shouts to you anywhere, any time, any place. She does have a preferred audience, preferring men to women, and never initiating contact with other children. She has an extremely limited range of things she likes to do, and many of them cause problems.

As I sit in the class, Naomi approaches me, not with 'Hiya' for once, but by turning round and backing up towards me. 'She wants to sit on your knee', interprets Joanne. She has an expectation that I want to know. I do, but I also like Joanne's assumption, the acceptance that this is something Naomi likes to do, which I should respect.

Some children like Naomi need to communicate, but they get so far and don't know how to go any further. One of Chairman Mao's sayings was, 'Destroy first, the rebuilding will take care of itself'. We know this doesn't make sense, but we still, too often, focus our attention on destroying established behaviour and working towards positive alternatives. Positive alternatives are fine as long term goals, but what should we do right now?

Naomi's behaviour is outside the limits acceptable in many situations – school (class, assemblies, mealtimes), home, at the shops. She's not amenable to conventional adult direction. She won't come when she's called, be quiet when she's asked, do what she's told, stop anything when told to.

Naomi loves to be chased, and to throw herself on the floor when she's about to be caught. She won't sit for long in the classroom, assembly or dining room, and this disrupts other children's learning. We can't simply accept disruption on the grounds of her limited understanding, because it does not respect other children's right to learning.

Naomi is noisy. She has a very limited range of words and sounds, but she uses them a lot. She recognises and greets a limited number of people excitedly and repeatedly – over and over. I happen to be one of them. In assemblies, for example, I often have to acknowledge her presence, replying 'Hiya', though a wave may suffice, to reassure her (?) and to allow the assembly to continue.

'Hiya' is not too much of a problem. It's a conventional word which she uses repeatedly, but at least in its accepted sense. The kissing poses more of a dilemma – at least for me. Unfortunately, she's not really happy with 'Hiya', she wants to pull me down for a kiss on the cheek and a sniff. Is this ethically OK? It's not the sort of thing I normally allow to happen, for a child's sake or for mine. Jill tells me: 'In class, we try to discourage this, by refusing to be dragged down by her. This was total rejection in her eyes, so we started to greet her first by putting our head close to hers, and taking the greeting to her'. Her need has been respected and moulded into something new.

In class, I watch as Naomi offers Karen an endless succession of useless gifts. Karen thanks her for each, 'Is that a present for me? Thankyou!', and more arrive. I look around at the language – all the adult language is to or about the children.

> **Jill:** We've introduced a communication board (cup, nappy, bells dish). Every morning she shakes the cup and shouts, so she always gets a drink – though she rarely wants one! But she enjoys the attention and reaction.

Naomi's educational programme is based on developing her communication skills through her favourite games – these are the games babies and parents love. Jill is becoming significant by having these games to offer. Jill describes the games – note that she describes them as activities rather than targets.

Naomi loves anticipation games. I sit directly opposite her with both chairs as close as possible with her knees inside mine. Jill matter of factly tells me Naomi tends to wreck the classroom – tipping things up, emptying cupboards, always looking for a reaction, and, ideally, to be chased. 'We usually just leave her to it because she will eventually run out of things to tip up.'

It's one of those decisions where 'creative ignoring' has been more effective in reducing the occurence than intervening to prevent.

We play 'Hold your hands up, count to three, tickle.' She'll raise her arms ready for this. I have sat for 45 minutes with Naomi and she has let me play with her like this. I'm sure she would have let me continue all day. She won't tolerate any outside involvement from others if they try to join in. She will push them away roughly shouting 'Aah' loudly at them – she's very good at expressing her anger! The focus here is on becoming significant to Naomi through the activity and the interaction. Get them right and Naomi will learn. In Class Six, Naomi is accepted, her interests and behaviour have been observed and understood. She is now no longer as desperate for constant attention – and she can take calmer attention for longer. She joins in with more activities, and can be approached by adults without being dragged into her kissing and sniffing routine every time.

Vanessa: Are we allowed this, Vanessa?

. . . in which staff show respect

Vanessa has some very fixed ways of behaving and of looking at the world. She is often desperate for something which appears to have no intrinsic value or meaning – a plastic number three, or an orange brick, for example. She's at that delightful stage where she makes mistakes like calling an orange brick an apple brick, but she's also learned that if she says 'Clown, clown, clown' for long enough, this will eventually produce results. These objects are important to her, and their importance is respected. She switches from theme to theme very quickly, and will soon become desperate for something else. There's negotiation over their availability, since she won't do much else when she has something like this to play with.

We regularly have live music in school, which she adores. I'm intrigued to see that she's often allowed to stand in front of the musicians, in ecstasy, when this would not be accepted from others. The idea that children don't respect different expectations proves unfounded.

Vanessa comes in to the class one morning, smiling, and walks straight up to the computer. She's greeted as she arrives, but she's not fussed, and she's allowed to play uninterrupted. She stays a while, then looks around. It's time to sit down at the table for the register. The table is established as a natural focus for more sustained and controlled activity. Equipment, adults, encouragement, other children, are all attractions. Vanessa is reluctant to sit with the others, but she's tempted. Karen spots this – 'She's coming' – she creates a space – 'Sit here, Vanessa'.

Vanessa eventually joins us at the table. Joanne watches her, 'Have you seen what she's done? She's not interested in the puzzle pieces – she just wants the empty tray!' This unconventional approach to jigsaws is accepted and respected because, from Vanessa's viewpoint, it's meaningful and constructive. Karen goes over to join in. She picks up a piece and asks, 'Are we allowed this, Vanessa?'

What progress has she made? Vanessa's problems are deep rooted and progress has been slow. She demonstrates an understanding of the world which we haven't yet tapped into, and she has now transferred to the TEACCH group for pupils with autism.

Carl: 'D'you want some help?'
. . . in which staff become significant by having something to offer

Carl's pre-admission reports were largely negative, describing 'considerable behaviour difficulties'. He nipped, thumped and bit other children, and was quickly frustrated if things didn't go his way. He was described as having 'a range of challenging behaviours including hair pulling, biting, hitting and smearing faeces'. A consultant's (brief) report told us he 'would benefit very little from education'.

But reading these reports, which often focus on challenging behaviour, is an art. As a school for children with learning difficulties we have to tease out why children display challenging behaviour even before they arrive. The behaviour may indeed be a reason for child to leave a mainstream environment, but it's not in itself a reason to come to our school. If, as is usually the case, the challenging behaviour seems to have clear origins in learning or communication difficulties, we may well be an appropriate placement.

With Carl it was obvious that his challenging behaviour was less of a problem than his difficulties in learning and communicating, and he came to us.

Sometimes Carl's signing was so extravagant and excited that he thumped someone. He discovered that this produced a more interesting response than when he signed into thin air. From the start the focus was on teaching Carl to sign more effectively. He did nip, scratch and bite, but not as much as we had feared, and his behaviour soon improved, as did his signing. By the time he came to Class Six, Carl had learned a great deal. He knew that adults are significant and helpful, can get you what you want, can be trusted, and are worth co-operating with.

I watch Karen and Carl engaged in a delicate negotiation about a jigsaw. Carl wants to complete the puzzle, but it's a challenge. He finds the pieces small and difficult to manipulate. I watch Karen prompt and support. Her expectation of co-operation is enough to keep him on task. 'Carl, pick them up', she prompts, as pieces fall accidentally. He watches her intensely. She continues, 'Come on, I'll help ya. Go on, you get that one', and he does. 'D'you want some help, Carl? Sit down, Carl', she prompts. He sits down and tries another piece.

Carl spots me, realises I'm not usually in his room, and points at me, smiling – a recognition of something out of the ordinary. This, he insists, is worth commenting on. Joanne leaves the room. He laughs and points to the door. She is a significant feature in his world and her absence is worth commenting on. He signs in the confident expectation of acknowledgement. Carl is working towards a target through spontaneously responding to a real event, not working his way through a language programme.

Carl now understands what is going on around him more clearly, and feels more useful in class. Carl loves approval and success. He claps himself, manipulates adults' hands to clap him, and bows when he judges that he has succeeded. We always suspected that Carl had good comprehension of spoken language. This year he has learned to act upon this knowledge without prompts. He now responds consistently to instructions such as 'Take the cup to David', or 'Pass me a paper towel'.

Carl's early attempts to communicate were hampered by his rough and ready approach to signing. We have built on his interest in people. Familiar staff have become important and significant to him. He now signs more proficiently, and has greater confidence in his ability to communicate. His signs are clearer, we are more familiar with his approximations, and he now believes in signing.

Children who have very little understanding of relationships or communication

Mark began to understand a little more clearly that people can express their wants and needs to one another.

Mark: 'Round and round the garden'
. . . in which staff become significant by having something to offer

Mark has learned a few skills – saying 'Hiya' and stroking hands, and seems to feel this is enough. Mark learned to say 'Hiya' several years ago. It's an appropriate greeting, and he says it in context. Unfortunately, he's never moved on from this – if anything, he now communicates less.

Mark's passivity is a real challenge. He has very little interest in communicating, and rarely displays any needs. Mark will show pleasure by smiling and laughing, but rarely shows fear, pain or distress – perhaps its a good way to live, but, unless we can help him communicate, he risks becoming a young person, and then an adult, whose needs are overlooked because he doesn't know he can express them.

A key issue in all human relationships is knowing what the other person wants. Mark presents great challenges to a teacher because, although there are things he likes, there's very little that he wants. Can we motivate him to want more? He won't learn to communicate until we can give him a reason to do so.

Setting targets for Mark is a delicate balance between acceptance and high expectations. It's tough with a child like Mark. There are quite a lot of things he likes to do, but he doesn't understand much about how to get them. So, he does like things which spin, and if he spots one he'll be off after it, but his real problem is not understanding that people can be used as a means to an end. Jill offers many of the things he likes – music, for example. In an environment which unconditionally offers music, Jill may help establish a link which leads to communication.

I like atmospheres like this, in which progress is likely to take place, in which you can sneak up on development, or let is sneak up on you. If you're focusing on the environment and relationships, targets and expectations can be more fluid and responsive than those we write at an annual review – important though they are.

Thus the comment I hear one morning, 'He's never done that before', communicates an observation and assessment, reports to colleagues, raises expectations, monitors and rewards progress. Having to write things down does focus the minds of those who need the structure, does encourage a consistent approach, and enables them to monitor and evaluate practice, but, in the end, paperwork's only real advantage is its longevity.

Behaviourism has been a powerful influence on special education for many years. Its appeal is its directness, simplicity and structure. Though the excesses of the 1970s are over, its influence is now enshrined in law, as it is integrated into the US derived model of Individual Education Plans (IEPs). We must remember that this is not the only way to organise children's learning. (Goddard 1997)

Conventional wisdom dictates that targets are written in terms of child behaviour. These can be useful, but we do need to be clear about the assumptions we make when we write a behavioural target – that we can predict how and what a child will learn. It's far easier to predict and plan how we will behave. There's a lot to be said for writing targets for adult rather than child behaviour. We should ensure that we give enough attention to things we can directly influence – namely our behaviour and the environment we offer. The ACL model suggests we concentrate on creating conditions and offering activities in which learning is likely to take place.

These are considerations for every sphere of education and training, but particularly pertinent for pupils with PMLD, where learning is very slow and unpredictable, and progress can be ephemeral. Mark will always learn slowly. Much of what we want him to learn does concern his challenging behaviour, since his experiences will be limited if he is perceived as disruptive. We want him to learn the social skills which will give him access to a wider range of experiences. He needs to learn to do something other than mouth whatever is in his hand, and to stay with a group of people or an adult through increased awareness of and interest in others. These are skills best learned in the context of social activity.

Mark likes music – especially 'Round and round the garden'. He will rotate his hands in a 'wind the bobbin up' motion. He loves the tumble drier in the next class, and toys that go round. Mark has now learned to sing some familiar tunes, and he will stay with a group for longer. Though he still appreciates the effect of a good tip, he no longer empties everything he can onto the floor. He has learned to operate simple switch toys – he specially likes those which go round like a washing machine, which would probably be his first choice as a toy. What has been offered has been what he wants.

Just after writing the above I went to a music festival with Mark's class. As I sat beside Mark I felt him pull my hand towards him, then press his finger into my palm. A flash of recognition – he was asking me to play 'Round and round the garden' – the first time in the years we have known one another that he had ever asked me for anything!

Children who have learned to communicate and relate through disruptive behaviour

Communicating by challenging adults can be very effective in gaining – or avoiding – adult attention. We discovered that David needed a more formal approach. Imtiaz already knew that thumping people kept them from making demands; he learned that moving his arms in a different way (we call it signing) could get him what he wanted. We learned that John needed to be in a different class.

David:

. . . in which staff implement an individual behaviour plan

David bursts in to the room, banging on the door to attract everyone's attention, signing 'Bus?' extravagantly. He's not rebuked for distracting everyone, or for asking about the bus, as he will throughout the day. Everyone's glad to see him, and his question is treated with the respect it deserves. 'No, we're not going on the bus today', responds Jill. In fact, every child comes in to class expecting a response – and getting one.

David can't stay still for long. He's always hot and sweaty, whatever the weather. In a way that's hard to put your finger on, he's not at ease with himself. David loves adult attention, he's especially keen to be chosen for jobs, such as taking the register and giving out drinks. He can do these well – he knows which children will take a biscuit off the tray and who needs the biscuit giving to them.

David is brighter than most of the rest of the class, and his behaviour is more consciously challenging. He copies other children's inappropriate behaviour – tipping chairs, throwing things, interfering with other children's activities. He spits and smacks children and adults. This is not consistent with what we would expect from a child of his ability. Though one of the characteristics of this class is acceptance and respect, the approach to David's behaviour demonstrates how staff discriminate between children.

I have put a great deal of emphasis on acceptance and on informal relationships, perhaps suggesting a lack of structure. Nothing could be further from the truth. The structure is deep and complex because it's embedded in the ethos, not rooted in the paperwork. But sometimes this is not enough. How do the staff react when a child doesn't respond to this approach? David is accepted and welcomed for himself, but some of his behaviour isn't. Being bitten or thumped is never pleasant, but is far less acceptable from David than from Imtiaz – he does know better. It was decided that a more formal approach was required. This meant writing an individual behaviour plan or IBP. Should a child have an IBP? We assume that if a teacher feels one might be appropriate, they are probably right. Why might a teacher feel this?

If a child's behaviour is causing problems despite the application of the usual repertoire of rewards and sanctions:

- the use of restraint is considered appropriate – we address this sensitive issue directly;
- the teacher wants to implement a particular approach.

IBPs have several practical benefits:

- The process ensures a range of adults working with a child discuss a problem. This often clarifies issues, leads to new approaches, encourages consistency, leads to advice from further afield and ensures we involve parents.
- The pressure on a teacher is eased. The message to the teacher is: 'We've all talked about this problem – you're doing what we agreed was the thing most likely to succeed'. The responsibility is on the group to come up with new ideas, not on the teacher to succeed as if by magic.
- Where there is an ethical issue, e.g. restraining a violent pupil, or one who wants to run in the road, the responsibility for addressing that issue is taken away from the teacher and shared by the group/school/LEA. The child (and the parents, the headteacher, the LEA), is protected from unethical practice.

In these circumstances, it's essential for the teacher, as well as the child, that approaches are written down.

IBPs don't guarantee freedom from abuse or malicious or mistaken allegations, but they do provide a significant degree of protection for all concerned, and do allow actions to be questioned objectively and in a non-threatening manner.

Our IBPs are short and to the point. We outline specific behaviour we are concerned about, the problems this leads to, and describe a very clear response. This is one of the occasions when a behavioural approach can help by being very specific, objective and clear enough for all who work with a child to try to implement.

David persisted in anti-social behaviour, particularly spitting and smacking, throughout the year, and a more formal approach is still in place. David now behaves acceptably for longer, and communicates more effectively, but his anti-social behaviour problems are deep rooted, and still cause problems.

Imtiaz: 'Sweetie, please, biscuit.'

. . . in which staff defuse and use challenging behaviour

Imtiaz finds people usually respond when he throws things or kicks them.

In Class Six one morning, I am scribbling down what I see. I look around the room – the floor is covered in equipment and toys. 'Shall we tidy up and do the register?' suggests Jill. 'Imtiaz – come for the register.' He puts his feet up to swing a kick. Jill laughs, and picks him up fondly. 'Do you want to take this register back?' She offers a deal, 'Stay here and you can take it. Sit here'. He responds assertively, signing 'Biscuit, biscuit', and banging the table. Jill's impressed with his signing: 'Imtiaz, he's so cute, isn't he?' Imtiaz continues to sign: 'Sweetie, please, biscuit!'

Later, Imtiaz has had several biscuits; Jill tells him there are no more for the time being. But he's after more. She comments on his persistence: 'He's so cheeky, Imti – he always asks for a bic when he's finished his work!' He goes across the room and begins to kick and thump equipment. Everyone's spotted him, but they all smile and ignore him. He continues to kick.

Jill follows Imtiaz to a quiet corner and sings 'Round and round the garden'. Imtiaz is upset because there's no sweet for him and the others are getting one. Karen asks: 'Why's he not allowed one?'

Imtiaz is one of the few children we have admitted to the school against my better judgement. Reports from nursery spoke of aggressive behaviour leading to the hospitalisation of staff and pupils. I believed young children at Millwood would be put at risk, and suggested the local authority look for an alternative placement, or, at least, additional staffing. But there was nowhere else, and staffing is our responsibility. So we took him, and moved him quickly up to be with older, less vulnerable children.

Jill tells me:

> 'The first time Imti let me near him was when I played Round and round the Garden. After I stopped he grabbed by hand to do it again. We all did this with him over and over again, as it was the first sign of Imti communicating a desire. It calmed him down and slowly we could get him to do other things – shape sorters, easy jigsaws, and looking at books.
>
> We deal with his aggression by not reacting to his threats or punches or kicks, by stroking the back of his neck, by leading him away from a situation without any recognition of his aggression.
>
> We also try to recognise what makes him angry – when he has a dirty nappy, when he can't get his own way, when he is unwell, especially with a bad cold, when he has trouble breathing or when his eczema is bad.
>
> Once a pattern of work was established, we introduced treats as a reward, and continued to sign to him. He quickly learned the signs for 'please', 'toilet' and 'biscuit'.

Sometimes Imti will flip for no reason – books and toys get slammed onto the floor. We can't identify anything that has triggered him off, but we can usually stop this by picking him up and sitting with him and so changing the situation.'

Imtiaz is still a very aggressive child, but he's not treated like one. He has made significant progress in his ability to communicate – he now has five signs he uses consistently. His aggression is more selective, but is never on the scale we read of in his pre-admission reports.

John:
. . . in which staff realise John is the odd one out

John suffered from lack of experience, but saw that Imtiaz got attention when he threw things, Vanessa when she flapped her arms. His attempts to get results through their methods produced mixed results – some attention, but John is bright enough to want more.

The first task of a class teacher is to design an environment in which children can learn. Each class has a potentially optimum environment, which takes into account the needs of the children, the staff and the available resources.

The most difficult classes are those with an odd one out. It doesn't really matter if that pupil is brighter or less able that the rest of the class, is challenging when the rest are amenable, or even is amenable when the rest are challenging. It's difficult to design an environment which takes this into account. So, a key issue in offering equal rights and opportunities and experiences is how to group pupils. We review and alter our methods of doing so in time for each September.

Let's get back to John. And make the point that he did not do well because he did not fit. John's lack of experience of social situations meant that in school he was trying to learn how people behave by watching his peers. Class Six did not provide appropriate models. If the cause of the challenges from John were rooted in the class, there was only one thing to do. We moved him as quickly as we could into another class. This was done with some reluctance, since we had hoped that John would provide a positive role model for other children, but he was swamped by their behaviour, and jealous of the attention they were able to get. Next door, with older and more able peers, he quickly settled down and began to model himself on the more positive behaviour he saw there.

Characteristics of the approach

This section describes the characteristics of the environment, which fosters positive behaviour, offers structure, is busy and active, is fun, and offers acceptance and respect. Within this environment, staff use professional detachment combined with human involvement, implement specific approaches to more intransigent behaviour, and knowingly use their personal styles.

The environment

What characterises this environment in which most children find themselves behaving in new and more fulfilling ways and communicating more effectively?

This is an environment which:

1. Fosters positive behaviour

This class hinges on creating an environment which fosters positive behaviour, in which positive behaviour becomes the norm, and leads to reward – especially social reward. It's structured on a belief that negative behaviour has been learned, and can be unlearned. The message is clear: 'I approve of you as a person, but I don't approve of what you are doing'.

2. Offers structure

Whenever I visit the class I am struck by the contrast between the outward chaos – toys and equipment everywhere – and the deep sense of calm, security and structure that comes from staff confident in their work, and children confident in the adults. In the midst of all this, there's always individual 1:1 work going on: Joanne and David drawing circles, seemingly oblivious to all around them; Karen working round a corner with another child, as a succession of children approach her with things to show or to offer her.

The structure comes from an environment which includes adults who are always available and behave predictably, a consistent routine, and accessible equipment.

3. Is busy and active

The room is always busy, and often untidy. Jill spots Imtiaz reading a book. She goes to sit beside him and guides him to sit beside her. They read the book together. Children move from activity to activity and approach adults and tasks confidently. Adults join children at their chosen activities and respond to approaches, encouraging children to join in other tasks. All children are active most of the time.

4. Is fun

There's a real sense of fun. Jill takes the cover off the computer, spots Naomi standing, unsure what to do next. Suddenly she finds Jill has popped the cover on her head. Why? It's an instinctive response, paralleling parent/infant play, interacting on a level appropriate to Naomi, and giving her a problem to solve. Naomi smiles and pulls it off.

5. Offers acceptance and respect

There's a sense of respect/acceptance/understanding/perspective that allows Vanessa to be left quietly to eat and drink, without adult interference. Naomi's constant greetings, Imtiaz's love of having his neck tickled, Mark's fascination for things which turn – all are respected as legitimate interests. Most requests, especially well-expressed ones, are respected and rewarded.

Approaches and techniques

This approach is based on professional detachment and human involvement with the ability and knowledge to use additional techniques when required.

Professional detachment

Observing and monitoring
How do the staff know what to do? All wait for, spot and create opportunities. They constantly monitor the situation, for themselves and each other. They instinctively report progress to one another in passing – 'She asked for blackcurrant, she usually asks for red pop'. This is real recording and reporting. All have an ability to attend to one child, accept approaches from another, and scan them all.

Hypothesising
They then relate their observations to their hypotheses about the children's behaviour – 'He's kicking the table because he wants a biscuit' – and act on them. Here's an opportunity to recognise an unacceptable request, and to use the opportunity to teach a more conventional way of asking for something.

Human involvement

Becoming significant by having something to offer
All the adults have developed different roles and responsibilities with individual children. It's the key worker principle, but less formal and more fluid, and it's based on the development of relationships, not on administrative convenience. They swap responsibility for children almost instinctively – if and when one struggles with a child, another takes over, interchanging roles and responsibilities. The staff become significant too by using their power as communicators. They work endlessly with their faces and voices, their presence and intuitive understandings, to be the most enjoyable and engaging things in the room.

Showing respect
A key issue in all human relationships is knowing what the other person wants. If you can offer this, you can, as the book says, win friends and influence people. This principle holds very true in Class Six. Although the children may be confused about what they want, and may want things we don't really want them to have, unless we start from their motivation rather than ours, we're going to have a struggle. What does Imtiaz want when he kicks? There's no doubt Vanessa sometimes needs, longs for, a plastic number three. We don't have to know why, though this might help, but we do have to respect that this is what she wants. To use these motivations as a reward is an obvious way in, but I have seen staff going much further, using the ostensible motivations – accepting and using them, turning them into something more productive. Thus, the class uses all sorts of

rewards – sweets, toys, time away from adult interference – this is what the child has developed, come with. These are accepted, but quickly moulded into something different, based on relationships and social rewards.

Approaches to more intransigent behaviour

Recognising the odd one out
When a child is clearly not making as much progress as we expect, we ask whether the environment is appropriate. If not, a move into another class, or school, may be required.

Implementing an Individual Behaviour Plan
If a child appears to be in an appropriate environment but still displays a significant degree of challenging behaviour, a more formal approach may be required. This involves meeting parents and other professionals to write an IBP, which may or may not involve using a behavioural approach.

Knowing how to defuse and use
To ignore challenges is textbook stuff, but it's only part of the story. To use the challenge is difficult but can be very effective. I've learned a great deal this year about how challenges can be respected as legitimate messages – mostly 'I want you' – and then turned into something positive. I've come to realise the limitations of ignoring the bad and rewarding the good. If you're really good, you can accept the bad and use it for good.

Naomi, for example, often passes my room on her way to the bathroom. She doesn't like to be directed, she doesn't like to walk far, and she is heavy. She's learned that she can effectively take over by throwing herself onto the floor. She also likes to run (away). Joanne and Karen know all this. They've turned the challenging behaviour of running into a game, dashing along the corridor with her to and from the bathroom. Is this a tale worth telling? I think it is, because most of us would approach the problem directly, asking, 'How can we make her get up?' In this example, staff use the knowledge they have of the world from the child's perspective, and use this to avoid the problem. And as time goes on, she is less likely to throw herself down. It's what you need versus what you want.

Staff knowingly using their personal styles
We struggled to distinguish between the individual teaching styles of Jill, Joanne and Karen. Their consistency is, in fact, a powerful tool. Jill is clearly the teacher, and takes the lead in planning away from the classroom, but within the classroom there is an equality which uses the strengths of everyone, and a closeness which gives an intuitive shared understanding of situations.

Everything which characterises good parenting is here, but with a subtle air of detachment which takes away guilt and increases objectivity. These are all warm, reliable and positive people who care about these children and their progress, and take a delight in their company.

They have a detachment which allows children space to play and experiment, but within a secure framework. They respect the children's physical space, but offer physical contact. They know who and when to leave alone.

Their spoken language prompts and supports the children's activities, never bombarding or dominating, often using motherese, always responsive to the child. They question, suggest and comment, but rarely explain, since this may impose an inappropriately adult perspective. Through their language they help children interpret and understand the world, and give them tools to express their own ideas.

Their body language signals acceptance and availability. They smile and touch, and seize opportunities to intervene, but pace their interventions carefully, taking cues from the child, moving on when the child needs peace, prompting when the child is stuck. Through body language which is calm, natural and unselfconscious, they transmit security and build up children's confidence in themselves and their abilities.

In summary, classroom equipment is almost incidental. The staff recognise themselves as the ultimate teaching tool.

When a child says no

Much of the success of the class lies in working around challenges, but what if the challenge is direct – a child who refuses to do something?

It's quite clear that this class succeeds through creating an environment in which incidents are reduced to a minimum. However, it's not a free for all. How, then do the staff deal with a child who just says 'No' when asked to do something? I asked Jill. She reminded me that no-one in Class Six actually verbalises 'No', but each is perfectly capable of letting you know they don't want to do what you ask.

The first principle comes from the practice of observing then hypothesising. A different approach is taken to each child, based on the knowledge the staff have of that child, and their beliefs about what it is reasonable to expect from him or her.

If Naomi refuses to do what she is asked, this is interpreted as making a choice – she has chosen to do something else. A confrontation is not appropriate. The refusal is not interpreted as challenging but is used as an opportunity to teach her that she can make choices by respecting her response.

Mark has little understanding of the nature or purpose of communication, he doesn't understand 'Yes', 'No', facial expression, body language or tone of voice. This is a major problem when he puts unsuitable (some of them very unsuitable) things in his mouth. It's inappropriate and dangerous to fish them out, so Jill decided to try to get the message across by packing as many modes of communication as she could into one package. 'I stood in front of him, with my face in front of his, and said 'No' very firmly. I signed 'No' and held out my hand'. To her surprise, Mark understood, and removed whatever was in his mouth. He began to do this consistently, and then with other members of staff. This was one of the first times he'd responded to an instruction.

Jill summed up their approach to David as follows. We make sure that anything we ask David to do is reasonable. He often refuses, but usually this is not because it's something he doesn't want to do, but to get a reaction. We repeat the request up to three times, then change our tone and facial expression. By this stage he begins to realise this is turning into an instruction, not a request. If he still refuses, we will physically prompt him. For example, if we want him to put a book away, we will close the book, ask him to pick it up, and if necessary, lead him by the hand to the cupboard.

Carl responds to facial expression – especially disappointment or dismay. When he's decided not to co-operate and he sees this reaction, he mimics our expression, and we can see him thinking, 'Oh no, I've dropped one here'. Carl responds to praise, so after he's completed the task – even if it took three instructions – we give him loads of praise.

Imtiaz often responds aggressively to an approach. I mentioned earlier that he's never given me the time of day. Jill explains how he rarely initiates an approach to anyone. What do they do when his body language says 'No'? We take him by the hand and lead him to things. We ask him to do something and he responds aggressively. It's easy to ignore him and not make demands on him because of this aggression. We work round this. If he won't do what he is asked we just take him by the hand and lead him but we do avoid getting involved in physical struggles. He loves the reaction and he knows who will react.

A management perspective

What does the school do to encourage the development of this way of working?

We work hard to create and maintain an atmosphere of acceptance and respect for all. This is not a sentimental or unrealistic establishment – part of an atmosphere of acceptance is to encourage and accept the expression of contradictory views. Nor is this is a staff of saints – it's a staff of motivated professionals, trying to do a difficult job well. This whole school philosophy, encompassing all members of the school community, encompasses all adults and, I believe, percolates down in several ways.

Staff are able to act confidently, to take their own decisions, talk frankly about problems, and their own perspective, and children are treated with respect. I hope this ethos of acceptance was one of the factors which allowed and encouraged this team to develop their own, very individual style.

A summary of the teaching style

How can we summarise this style of working?

This is an approach in which staff balance professional detachment which keeps them objective about the work they are paid to do every day, with a human involvement which is warm, caring and individual. They accept and observe the children, then offer and act on hypotheses about their behaviour. They have evolved a very specific style of working.

- They maintain a positive ethos. This is a very natural style. Staff are very relaxed with one another and with the children. It's seen in their language, 'Er, that's not yours, Flower', as something unsuitable is taken from Carl.
- They use an appropriate style of interaction for each child. This often echoes infant/caregiver interactions. We do believe in age appropriateness, and in the principle of Person First. We see ourselves, and like to be seen, as one of Bury's primary schools – it's the one which takes children with learning difficulties, but it is firstly a primary school. These are primary-aged children, but they still need input at a level they can access. So there is more physical contact and parenting than with most children of this age. This is reflected in facial expression, tone of voice, content and style of language, and softer body language. As a primary school, we're committed to giving children full access to the National Curriculum, in a way which puts judgements about children's needs as the single most important consideration when designing targets and activities – but that's a chapter in itself.
- They respect one another. All our classes have a class teacher and one or two NNEBs. Walk into any class and it might take some time to work out who is who. I think this is healthy – we need all staff to act as responsible professionals, making their own decisions within an overall framework. This includes interchanging responsibilities. In assembly, a child struggles on Karen's knee. Joanne instinctively takes over. Neither attaches much significance to this, but it's real professional teamwork. Members of this team respect one another professionally, and constantly tease each other socially.
- They minimise the prospect of challenging behaviour occurring. Staff recognise that attention is reward and so avoid giving incidents any more significance than is strictly necessary. They know that behaviour which is rewarded is repeated. This is one debt we owe to the behaviourists. Fortunately these three colleagues of mine lean instinctively to the Interactive Approach – it's probably their greatest gift. They have seen beyond the cliché of ignoring the bad and praising the good – they know how to defuse and use challenging behaviour.
- They do not allow record keeping to interfere with teaching. We keep paperwork to a minimum, asking staff to use their professional judgement to decide what is worth recording, within a whole school framework. But most assessment, recording and reporting happens verbally. Adult to adult language almost exclusively passes on important messages about children, as in 'He's never done that before!'

Conclusion

I am very aware of the inadequacy of this account. I write as an outsider who hasn't spent enough time in the class to fully understand what is going on.

I once made the mistake of overriding Karen's plans for Naomi. At a practice for a Harvest Festival I noticed Naomi was not included, she was left on a chair at the back of the hall. I should have attached more significance to the look of doubt which flashed across Karen's face as I suggested that Naomi shouldn't be left out, and led her by the hand to the table of gifts. She threw herself to the floor, crying, and pulling away from me. Karen came over to rescue the situation, and then spent the rest of the session calming her down. I hadn't really thought about what was going on. Karen knows Naomi much better than I do, and cares for her. She would have been part of the practice if it was going to work. I just upset her. I know better now!

The work is so subtle that I know there is much I have missed. It's not helped by the staff's self-effacing approach to their work. Like many people working with young children, they don't know how good they are. John Bowlby once described parents, especially mothers, as much maligned. The same is true of many of those who work with young children, particularly those working in special education, where we are frequently characterised by one of several equally erroneous descriptions: child minders, when we are working with those who are patently more difficult to teach than most, or dispensers of magic or, perhaps even worse, medical tricks, which will cure problems. We are none of these, we are simply educators. The staff in Class Six at Millwood School are supremely good at this. Though they do a difficult job very well, it's important to recognise that exceptional practice is happening in many other classes and in many other schools throughout the county. This just happens to be an opportunity to share some ideas and experiences.

The success of this class hinges on the creation of an environment which fosters positive behaviour, in which positive behaviour becomes the norm, and leads to (social) reward. The focus is on this, rather than on the elimination of behaviour which is challenging to adults, but self-perpetuating because it is rewarding to children.

Many readers may feel that this account describes common sense. That's what Karen, Joanne and Jill told me when they read early drafts of this chapter. My response is that this approach is based on sense, but it's not very common to see it done this well.

References

Emblem, B. and Frew, B. (1988) 'Drawing from life', *Times Educational Supplement* 23 September: 40.

Goddard, A. (1997) 'The role of individual education plans/programmes in special education: a critique', *Support for Learning* 12(4), 170–174.

Mesibov, G. B., Schopler, E., Hearsey, K.A. (1994) 'Structured teaching', in Schopler, E. and Mesibov, G. B (eds) *Behavioral Issues in Autism*, 195–207. New York: Plenum.

Nind, M. and Hewett, D. (1994) *Access to Communication: Developing the Basics of Communication with People with Severe Learning Difficulties Through Intensive Interaction.* London: David Fulton Publishers.

Chapter 5

Commentary: managing incident challenging behaviour – principles

Dave Hewett

Introduction

What is an incident?

The use of the term 'incident' implies a flexible concept. It is the period of time that the person is being very difficult to be with. This may often be a short, sometimes sharp period where some exciting and daunting things take place. We might also feel that some incidents actually last for much longer, sometimes days, with the person remaining at a heightened and probably disagreeable state of arousal, with occasional peaks occurring where she/he becomes even more disagreeable. I also like the term to imply those situations where it looks very much as if a person will provide a challenging situation, but then nothing really happens – the situation may have been effectively handled and defused.

Additionally, some people have a lifestyle and a way of behaving which has such a bad 'fit' with their environment and everyone around them that their life seems like an incident. These will often be people who are still at early stages of development, who have not yet learnt to relate and communicate well, whose conditions may also be characterised by extreme anxiety, particularly concerning social situations. Often, because of their abilities, they will not have adopted the way of behaving shared by most of the rest of us, but have developed instead highly personalised styles of behaviour to which huge energy and attention may be devoted.

I find it helpful, however, to think in terms of 'incidents' so there is a focus for staff on practice techniques which are applicable to these situations. It is none the less also vital not to conceptualise incident management practices as being too different from the style of staff behaviour generally. The two should of course be related, and influence and overlap each other. There should not be too much of a sense of a sudden 'clunk' as a person's behaviour hits a threshold and staff shift into incident management.

What is incident 'management'?

Here again, I find the thought of trying to 'manage' incidents to be a helpful concept. 'Managing' seems to be a realistic staff goal for some of the

69

complexities of the way people feel and behave. Sometimes we may only 'manage' to get through the incident, to cope, with nothing too terrible having happened. Having skills for 'managing' incidents seems to be a less absolute and demanding expectation than 'controlling' them. Looking to develop techniques for 'managing' seems to imply an orientation toward flexibility and imaginativeness in what staff actually do. Looking for good technique in incident management ultimately also implies that one can become just that – a good incident manager.

What should we do?

One of the hardest things for staff is to be faced, in the middle of the most demanding situation created by a person's behaviour, by the question, 'What on earth shall I do next?' This is the major issue for staff on a daily basis when working with people who can be difficult. When students/clients are being challenging, we need to know what to do, how to handle it and – crucially – the background or framework of workplace values, attitudes and policies that gives guidance about what to do in difficult situations.

The contributors to this book all give advice about these matters in various ways. There is clear, practical advice on things to do in situations. These practicalities are usually related to a workplace ethos and a set of guiding principles, and sometimes further related to the employer's written policy. Not all employers have policies, but the good ones aim to give guidance to staff on practice and technique in difficult situations. There are examples of staff sitting and talking, evaluating and thinking together, and taking the results of this work back into the difficult situations they face. This reflection enhances the framework of thought and action which individual staff may call upon to help them.

Naturally, in selecting contributors to this book, my own preference for values and practices has been paramount. I have asked for accounts of their work from people who have practices and values of which I broadly approve. This does not necessarily mean that I could be called upon to endorse every behaviour that individual staff indulge in, but that their principles of practice, and those of their employers, are humane and down to earth, conforming to the general style which I would normally advocate. Martin Bertulis puts this well (Chapter 2) when he points out that the descriptions of incidents given by his staff may not be 'perfect practice', but he is none the less clearly proud of the staff attempts to reach the best possible practice by adhering to a set of principles and values and by ongoing, honest reflection.

The principles and practices exemplified by the contributors, and those set out in this chapter, broadly conform to the noticeable trend in working practices nationally over some years. Generally, employers are sending staff the message that the style of work they require with people who can be challenging should be based on understanding, humanity, respect and empathy. These values will be the basis of staff practices that are controlled and ordered, as gentle as possible, while still being as effective as possible in controlling and structuring the person's behaviour – showing them how to behave.

One of the principles of practice shown in the contributions to this book is the reality that it is necessary to base your practice in difficult situations, moment by moment, on working from a set of principles. Many staff, understandably, want to be told exactly what to do when 'this' or 'that' happens. This can be achieved up to a point, and the more effective teams talk about and/or write sensible guiding procedures for known recurring situations. However, expecting to be absolutely and precisely instructed in all of the behaviours that you as a member of staff will need in a situation is generally a mistake. It is more realistic and effective for staff to carry with them in their heads a set of principles for managing difficult situations. The principles offer a framework of decision making throughout the incident, but it is necessary to make judgements and decisions based on these principles and the existence of any helpful known procedures.

This type of approach is well evidenced in the work described by Nicki Bond and Don O'Connor (Chapter 3). They also clearly show how demanding it is for individual members of staff to be working in this way. It necessitates an attitude to managing people's behaviour where the staff cognitive processes – the decision making and judgements necessary – are looked upon as an interesting, enjoyable and natural aspect of the work. It demands that each individual member of staff thinks, reflects, talks. It can seem much harder than the obvious route of members of staff confronting 'bad' behaviour with powerful behaviour. Additionally of course, in order to operate guided by a set of working principles, it is necessary to think clearly in those situations, and therefore have sufficient internal calm.

This chapter sets out a framework of principles for the style of working in challenging situations illustrated by the contributors. The list in the next section has been compiled using some of the processes mentioned above: by learning from experience and from colleagues with better practices, by talking and reflecting, by reading and being aware of trends in the field of work with people with learning difficulties, particularly the thought and discussion in recent years on matters of personal rights. It is worth re-iterating again that working in the way advocated here can never be a universal panacea. People are complicated, it takes time for them to change their behaviours and the feelings which underlie them, and having good incident management practices is just one aspect of helping the person to progress and move on. Many challenging situations may end up being barely coped with rather than totally and effectively resolved, no matter what good practices staff may have. Indeed, a sensation of failure in some situations is to be expected (this is one of the principles given).

Principles of the sort set out here are often described as 'non-confrontational' in guidance documents or relevant literature. I prefer to avoid using the term though, strictly speaking, it is accurate. I have met staff who may well need a great deal of guidance, who equate non-confrontation with not doing anything much about the person's behaviour – even not intervening. They seem to operate a semantic confusion between 'intervening' and 'confronting'. Others maintain that non-confrontation is about 'letting people get away with it'. It must always be emphasised that using principles of non-confrontation is not about not doing anything or failing to act or intervene. It is not an easy option. There is an absolute dedication here to making judgements at all times about what would be an effective intervention during an incident of challenging behaviour – the intervention doesn't have to be a competitive confrontation.

Using these principles should not prevent staff from, to use some popular phrases, 'being firm,' helping people to 'control their behaviour', 'describe boundaries' for them, help them to have 'discipline' and know the 'consequences' of their actions. However, use of these principles pays very careful attention to the style of staff behaviour by which these things may be achieved. I hope it can be seen that all contributors illustrate this orientation to exerting external control.

A less emotively loaded phrase to describe these principles is 'interventions in incidents of challenging behaviour which attempt to avoid needless conflict'. There is an immediate implication here that the principles are intended to help staff to avoid viewing incidents of challenging behaviour as conflict situations that they must 'win' and that 'winning' them has an obviously beneficial effect on the sensibilities of the person with the challenging behaviour who loses.

A word here about human conflict. It would be silly to suggest that being involved in conflicts, sometimes winning them, sometimes losing them, is not a useful, natural and healthy human experience on occasion. However, if, as a service-user, this regular involvement in conflict is the style by which your behaviour is routinely managed, then this is indeed unhealthy.

I have the presumption that however dedicated staff may be to the avoidance of conflict, occasional conflicts nonetheless arise. For staff working with people with learning difficulties, so much of their job is concerned, rightly, with 'goal-blocking'. This means that it is a natural part of the job to restrict people's freedom to do what they want, for good reasons – safety and security, the needs of a group over-riding an individual's needs or desires, the necessity to follow a structure and timetable at times when individuals have other intentions. This aspect of the job can naturally give rise to open conflict, but actually most staff everywhere are good at achieving goal-blocking of individuals' wants or desires, most of the time, without it becoming open conflict. The occasional open conflict that does arise will probably give the person all of the experience of conflict that is healthily necessary, without the need for the staff to use the winning of conflicts as the style by which the person is routinely managed.

There is a further fundamental danger which arises from people with learning difficulties being routinely managed by the use of confrontation. Often I meet staff groups who work with adults and who may have attempted to control a person's behaviour by direct confrontation and by winning conflicts. Unfortunately, they find it to be impossible with this person – the staff routinely lose these competitions. The essence of the difficulties the staff face seems to be simply that the service user is better at it. The service-user has probably been around for a long time, been in care in many different places and met many staff, and, because of the nature of her/his behaviour, has accrued a wide and varied experience of conflict situations. She/he has developed good skills for these situations and rehearsed the use of them many times. This person may find confrontations an interesting and fulfilling experience where she/he can indulge the conflict expertise developed, and is prepared to commit more time and energy to the situation than the staff. Ultimately, the service-user is prepared to do things and take the situation further than the staff are prepared to. The staff are then faced with the painful process of backtracking in their style to find other ways of managing incidents with that person.

Actually, much of the above can apply to quite young service-users too. In my mind it does invoke the need to give particular attention to styles of behaviour management in the early years, to work very hard to develop the person's sense of human participation and co-operation, rather than operating models of domination and compliance simply because the person is tiny and seemingly susceptible. Bernard Emblem (Chapter 4) writes about a group of staff operating this priority. Rosemary Hawkins' work with Ann (Chapter 11) shows a small staff team dedicating themselves to it. Her account also illustrates the reality of the time and effort that is required and the ups and downs which can be experienced.

General principles for managing incidents of challenging behaviour

The list of general principles is set out in Figure 5.1, but it is not exhaustive. Teams working together may well wish to add to it and refine it, though for a list of principles, brevity is seen as a virtue. It is offered here as a framework for good practice in challenging situations, reflecting the work of the people in this book who have described their experiences. Each item in the list will be enlarged upon in turn. As principle 6, 'Have incident management techniques based on these priorities', brings with it the most content for the practicalities of incident management techniques, Chapter 9 is dedicated to it.

Though a 12-point list, it is hoped that the items are straightforward and practical enough for them to be remembered and carried in the mind while working. Principles 1 and 2 are seen as the most important. Indeed, I believe I have worked with staff who worked well simply from basing their practice on principle 1, stay calm, and 2, avoid contributing to the seriousness of the situation with your behaviour. The effect was that their practice more or less fell into line with the rest of the principles because they were operating principles 1 and 2 thoughtfully and creatively.

Principle 1: stay calm and have calm and/or ordered behaviour

It's so simple isn't it? Just stay calm no matter what you are confronted with and things will be better. Of course this is absolutely true, and surely no-one would deny the need to carry out this item of technique effectively. Good incident management depends on thinking clearly, and the less calm you are, the harder it is to think clearly.

In fact, it could be said that not only is this downright common sense, actually the employers *demand* of staff that they remain calm in their work. It simply isn't all right for members of staff to lose a grip on their own emotions, particularly anger and frustration, and work on with anger and frustration as the driving force. It does happen of course, but if anything particularly untoward happens to a service-user because a member of staff has 'lost it', the disciplinary consequences could be considerable. That was true even in the past when practices were less considered and more casual. I can remember experiencing workplaces where huge displays of powerful, angry behaviour from staff were commonplace, and well, just one of the things that happened. None the less, ultimately it would still have been a disciplinary matter if someone had, for instance, been injured as a result.

---

1. Stay calm and attempt to have calm and/or ordered behaviour.

2. Avoid contributing to the seriousness of the incident with your behaviour.

3. Get your priorities right:
   1. manage the incident
   2. work for an effective outcome rather than a winner and a loser.

4. Have incident management techniques based on these priorities.

5. Attempt to see the situation from the other person's point of view.

6. Assess and keep assessing.

7. Tune-in and stay sensitive to the other person's signals of arousal.

8. Maintain control of your own communication style and physical presence.

9. Have prepared mental structures for helping you to think and act.

10. Use time effectively and creatively.

11. Use teamwork.

12. Don't expect to manage all incidents successfully.

Figure 5.1 Some general principles for managing incidents of challenging behaviour at all levels of intensity and severity

It can be difficult to maintain calm in the face of much of the challenging behaviour that staff attempt to manage. However, the expectation that members of staff will achieve this is the right one. It is right for employers (and by implication the society we all serve) together, of course, with the service users, to expect that staff practices will be thoughtful and reasonable – *especially* in the most difficult circumstances. Members of staff do not have the right to lose their 'rag' because a person with learning difficulties behaves in ways which are difficult, naughty, obstinate, obsessive, violent, abusive, destructive, and so on. People with learning difficulties have the right to expect that staff will attempt to understand and empathise, to avoid blaming them for their behaviour or holding them solely responsible for it. They have the right to expect that even in the most difficult circumstances caused by their own behaviour, they will be dealt with by a person who is in control of her/himself, whose approach to their needs at those moments is methodical and ordered.

However, we need to be clear that people who become involved in work with people with learning difficulties are unlikely to be more saintly than others. They may have all sorts of fine qualities and outlooks that have brought them to the work, but an unusually effective 'internal gadget' for controlling feelings probably won't be one of them. Any member of staff must be prepared to recognise the very human experience of starting to lose your grip on yourself and have some procedures prepared for it. A few such procedures would be:

- Be honest and get to know your own internal signals that you are losing yourself.
- Be prepared to walk away. Losing the 'battle' is probably not as bad as losing yourself. Live to think and work during the next incident. There will probably be another even if you 'win' this one.
- Walking away is frequently not possible. Have therefore, or be prepared to work toward, the teamwork ethic that it is good practice to hand over to a colleague. This will not be a loss of 'face' or be seen as not managing – it is good practice. It is often particularly good practice during long and difficult incidents for two or more members of staff simply to relay each other.
- There may be routine occasions when colleagues are not available to you. Remain prepared to walk away if it is possible. If it is not possible, put extra work into developing your own techniques for remaining calm (see later).

Furthermore, it is as well to appreciate that the challenging behaviours produced by service-users can indeed produce all sorts of feelings in members of staff. Frustration and anger are likely to be common reactions, but occasionally feelings can include hatred (usually temporary) or a desire to be violent (or something) in return. It is probably best not to be too hard on oneself when this happens, it is an understandable reaction to difficult circumstances. It is wise to have available opportunities to vent these feelings appropriately – with trusted colleagues or a loved one who will not report your professional indiscretion – perhaps by attacking a pillow with a baseball bat or something similar. Indeed, recognising feelings and expressing them somehow is healthy and, ultimately, will surely contribute to calmness when in a difficult situation. In a sense these feelings are legitimate – they occur for good, understandable reasons and are unavoidable. The practice issue is that a member of staff must not allow these feelings to drive practice. Practice must be driven by reason and rationality.

Part of the art is to also acknowledge that absolute calmness in terms of complete mental serenity may not be possible. What is needed is some sort of knowing compromise. It is necessary to develop enough inner composure to keep ordered behaviour on the outside, while still experiencing, but managing, feelings such as frustration, anger, anxiety and even fear. Indeed, it might be advisable not to totally banish feelings such as fear, especially when dealing with the more serious incidents of violence. Fear can be a healthy thing to experience, it can assist one to guard against over-confidence, it can keep mental systems nicely on edge, and it can make sure that you devote the proper attention to a serious situation. Of course, too much fear and anxiety can be debilitating – there is a balance to be struck.

It is important to look upon the ability to be calm as a skill, a matter of technique which can be developed and enhanced. In a sense it is the most basic and crucial technique for good incident management practices. It is very difficult indeed to carry out all other techniques if this one is not successfully in place. The technique can be developed, it is not something inherited genetically. Of course, you may have colleagues who seem naturally and annoyingly good at keeping their cool. There are many people like this and they are very fortunate people. They seem to have a natural ability to be calm because of all sorts of factors in the development of their personality and emotional make-up. Although these colleagues may be annoying, learning everything one can from them can help to develop personal technique. Even though they might have very low personal trigger thresholds and arousal levels, they may also have some very effective thoughts and attitudes which they bring to situations and which can be 'borrowed'. Some further ideas on the technique of calmness are outlined in Figure 5.2.

Furthermore, it is important not to take the issue of calmness to extremes. People who have learning difficulties do not necessarily need to be taught or cared for by calm robots. It is important that they also experience seeing staff who have feelings, problems, and ups and downs. Bernie Hunt (Chapter 6) describes the way in which her colleague, Peter, has a wide variety of natural behaviour he freely indulges at work. But he also has the technique to know and make judgements about the right personal style for different situations.

Principle 2: avoid contributing to the seriousness of the incident with your behaviour.

Some people are naturally very good at carrying out this principle. They are likely to be the ones who are also naturally good at keeping calm. However, there are many, many members of staff who may actually be relatively volatile

Give proper attention to yourself
Try to think about yourself. You are the most important person present. In particular it can be helpful to give attention to breathig, making sure that you give yourself proper amounts of oxygen. Some people have deliberate breathing exercises which they practice and can use subtly even in the most demanding of situations.

Continuously monitor your own arousal levels
Keep on checking with yourself as to how 'frustrated/angry/upset am I feeling'? Naturally, employ self-control, but try to recognise when self-control is becoming too rigid and brittle. Try to be aware when reason and rationality are being lost.

Have agreed procedures for when you are 'losing yourself'
As outlined in the previous section, be prepared to hand over or relay with colleagues and recognise this as good practice. Don't stay put when you are close to losing control of yourself.

Think positively
Try to have thoughts such as:
'This will end', 'this is what I am here for', 'it is my job to help this person'.
'Challenging behaviour is normal – this is part of the job.'
'It is understandable that this person has challenging behaviours.'
This incident is actually an interesting aspect of my interesting job.'

Think ahead
'What are my options for the next 30 seconds?'
'This will end.'
'I am prepared to hand over to a colleague if I have had enough.'

Have a mental 'quiet place'
Many people do this. Relaxation exercises at other times help with the development of a mental 'quiet place'. This mental image can be used even at the height of crisis.

Know you have technique
It is tremendously reassuring to know that you have a range of tried and trusted techniques for handling incidents, especially when you are feeling that you have not yet used all of them. This item may well be the hardest one to achieve, it takes work, experience, thought and discussion, perhaps reading.

Know that you are prepared
Have the reassurance that all practical preparation has been carried out.

Figure 5.2 Being calm during an incident of challenging behaviour

personalities themselves, but who have learnt to conduct themselves in challenging situations in line with this principle.

I worked with a colleague who seemed to have quite magical abilities to defuse some quite dreadful situations, simply by use of herself – her presence, her voice, her body language. When pressed to describe how she intervened with such apparent deftness, she thought hard for a while and then pronounced her guiding motto: 'I sort of continuously try and do the least to achieve the most'.

Such wisdom! This person had developed a fine art of awareness. She remained aware of her own inner processes and outward behaviours, she was continuously monitoring the aspects of her own behaviour that she was putting into the situation in an effort to manage it, and she stayed continuously sensitive to the positive or negative effects of her own behaviour on the person she was trying to manage. By this ongoing process of inward and outward reflection, she was often able to do the absolute minimum to be successful in incidents of challenging behaviour. Thus she achieved the desirable state of affairs of having a less stressful personal working life than the rest of us might.

None of this was at odds with her desire as a teacher to have order, to have people behaving well and respectfully toward each other, to get the students doing things that she wanted them to do and which she and colleagues judged to be beneficial for them. In that sense, she was as dedicated as any other teacher to having a 'disciplined' atmosphere where these features applied. She was actually a good 'goal-blocker'. Students did not get their own way all of the time with her, she did not shy away from imposing her own limits on their behaviours, or from preventing them from doing or having things which would be disruptive to order at that moment. However, she was good at being a 'goal-blocker' who did not provide the student with needlessly negative experiences. She simply recognised that it was possible to have all those things without being the controller and dominator of the environment, the most powerful person present in terms of behaviour. She also totally accepted that however good her general classroom management was, every day would produce some very challenging incidents and they had to be accepted and managed appropriately.

For all staff, one of the most classic 'mistakes' is to put too much of one's own behaviour into a challenging incident. Let's be fair to ourselves, making this 'mistake' is so easy to do, it is understandable, we are all only human. Getting it right can take time and it is unlikely that any person can ever be perfect at it. Getting it right relates fundamentally to the two aspects of principle 3 in the next section concerned with priorities: firstly, concentrate on managing the incident effectively, nothing else is as important; and secondly, work for an effective outcome to the incident rather than a winner and a loser. Two aspects of the inner processes of staff are likely to be major contributors to getting it wrong:

1. Practice issues: not having the right priorities, not monitoring one's own behaviour and its effects so that you know when you have done 'enough'.
2. Emotional issues: not being conversant with the 'personal limitations' one is likely to bring to difficult situations, not having sufficient ability to stay

calm, i.e. getting one's own emotional stuff tangled up in someone else's.

Item 1 will be dealt with in detail within the content of principle 3, get your priorities right, and principle 7, tune-in and stay sensitive to the other person's signals of arousal. Item 2 is concerned with tough personal issues for staff. It is significantly linked with the staying calm issues of the previous section, but also goes further into areas of personal introspection. To work successfully in challenging incidents, one needs some sort of conscious familiarity with one's own emotional processes and to guard against them becoming activated. A nurse I met briefly in a long-stay hospital summed this up with great wisdom and conviction: 'So often, it has been my own personal limitations that have got me drawn into conflict situations I didn't need to be in'.

Every member of staff is, of course, a personality with feelings, memories, attitudes, values, beliefs and personal mind-sets. All of these will be affecting the way that the person operates in a difficult situation. Some of these effects will be beneficial, e.g. positive values and attitudes positively affecting practice; and some will be not be beneficial, e.g. a person with a precarious emotional set-up quickly becoming an angry member of staff in a challenging situation. These are the personal limitations that one is likely to bring into the situation. The main idea is to try not to get your own feelings confused with the situation – the situation is about someone else's feelings. The difficulty is knowing about personal limitations, objectively identifying them and realising how and when they are likely to 'come on line' in your processes and behaviour. Here are some examples of things which are likely to be personal limitations; some of the items on the list are things which might, on the face of it, be seen as positive, correct or even noble, however, they still might operate as personal limitations:

- being a very angry or frustrated person on the inside;
- having an absolute dedication to justice and fair play;
- having a general sense of frustration about one's own performances in life generally;
- striving for perfection in everything you do;
- having an absolute desire for peace, order, tidyness, cleanliness;
- disliking people who behave 'badly';
- having the attitude that 'bad' behaviour is never acceptable;
- having the attitude that all sorts of behaviour is acceptable;
- viewing oneself as a very powerful personality – no-one gets the better of me;
- being likely to be easily offended.

Anger and frustration are likely to be the most common limitations we are all likely to bring to challenging situations, but they can be triggered into use by a variety of attitudes, beliefs and outlooks on life which are apparently contravened by the person's behaviour.

Becoming conversant with one's own personal limitations may not be easy. My former colleague was a lucky person who actually did not have too many. She was not complacent, however, and was able to describe objectively the amount of self-reflection she undertook at various times to keep herself in 'good shape' for her job. The nurse I met went on to describe her own personal journey from being an angry immediate intervenor in unjust, unacceptable behaviour, to becoming a more methodical practitioner who assessed the situation, her own processes and operated with a more ordered style. She related the amount of thought she finally started putting in to her inner anger and the way it boiled into other people's situations. She began to realise how often her own feelings got mixed up in situations and became one of the driving forces of them. She had embarked on a difficult-seeming process of talking about these things with colleagues, relating to them the realisations she was having about her own difficulties. She was pleasantly surprised to find that some of her colleagues empathised with relief, and 'personal limitations' became a topic for discussion amongst the team. These discussions she felt, had fundamentally contributed to the worth of individual team-members' practice and to team-working processes. She felt that the best thing she had done was to start to talk about it and to share the problem.

Principle 3: get your priorities right

Priority 1: manage the incident – other considerations are less important

This priority is easier to put into operation with the very severe incidents. When a person is right on the verge of awful destructiveness or violence, and if the person is large with powerful demonstrations of threatening behaviour, this tends to work well in clearing one's mind of the clutter of things like 'this person is in the wrong and deserves to be told-off'. But not always. Even in such situations, some staff may feel a compulsion, perhaps driven by personal limitations, to remonstrate, to punish, to bring the consequences of the person's behaviour to their attention, to show the person that staff cannot be 'pushed around'. All of these things may be justifiable and legitimate viewpoints, but the middle of an incident is not the right time to air them. It will probably result in staff putting more of their own behaviour into the situation than is needed. During an incident, the priority is to manage it and achieve an effective outcome – everything else can wait. This is especially true of major and serious incidents, but it is also a good principle to apply to minor ones. Many minor incidents can become major ones through the input of too much adverse staff behaviour.

In any event it is wise to consider the degree that the person being challenging is in a condition to carry out positive learning during the incident. People who are being challenging are normally experiencing emotional arousal – anger, distress, anxiety, fear, etc. As will be illustrated in Chapter 9, one of the incident management techniques is to make judgements about the person's arousal and respond accordingly. During increasing arousal people become less reasonable and rational. It is indeed possible to say and do quite a lot with people who are in lower states of arousal but, for instance, the decision to tell them off is a judgement to be made, not an absolute rule.

All of this relates to the ethos of the workplace and individual attitudes of members of staff. It relates to where the working practices lie on a continuum between, to put it crudely, controlling/punishing/dominating and communicating/understanding/defusing. The contributors to this book tend toward the latter end of the continuum in their practices and beliefs. None of them, however, display a *laissez-faire* attitude toward behaviour – they do attempt to control, order and achieve better behaviour. It also relates to the extent to which people with learning difficulties who have challenging behaviours might be viewed as responsible for their behaviour and capable of controlling it, given their present abilities and personal resources.

Priority 2: work for an effective outcome rather than winners and losers

An effective outcome is a simple thing: everyone calmed down, nobody hurt, nothing broken, nobody too traumatised, order restored. In the best of worlds this should be the only objective of incident management. As outlined earlier, it is possible to be directive with a person who is judged to be at a lower level of arousal and has abilities which make it worth while. However, the uncluttered thinking for staff which goes with the operation of this priority is a thing much to be cherished. There is here an implicit recognition that the service user will learn best when having fewer challenging incidents at other times. There is an implicit dedication to doing the least to achieve the most, and adopting the straightforward practices which go with it. There is also a dedication to avoiding a behaviour management style which is dependent upon the staff 'winning' situations and the services user 'losing' them.

Principle 4: have incident management techniques based on these priorities

Chapter 9 sets out practical advice for the sorts of techniques for incident management illustrated by the contributors to this book and in line with the principles advocated in this chapter. Once again, however, it is stressed that what is on offer there is a framework for further thought, discussion and action. Reading Chapter 9 will not equip a member of staff for every eventuality which will be encountered. It will not tell you exactly what to do in all situations. The practices outlined there will need to be thought about further, modified, refined and applied flexibly.

Principle 5: attempt to see the situation from the other person's point of view

In Chapter 1 there is discussion of the factors that may be contributing to a person's challenging behaviour. Part of the purpose of viewing what is happening to the person in this way is to develop systematic empathy and understanding. If we carry out an exercise of assessing and writing down all of the likely factors which contribute to the way a person behaves, it can be a significant lesson. It can then give a member of staff some extremely helpful thoughts and attitudes, such as: 'It's not surprising that this person has challenging behaviour – she/he should have'; 'It's silly of us to expect that this person will not have challenging behaviour'; 'Challenging behaviour is normal and natural for people who have difficulties with life such as these'.

These thoughts and attitudes are likely to contribute to the member of staff remaining more calm during the challenging incidents and operating with a foundation of empathy and compassion. It may then be all the more possible to project in one's incident management style the message to the person: 'Look, this behaviour is not alright, but I really do realise where you are coming from'.

Principle 6: assess and keep assessing

It is very important to base incident management practices moment by moment on an objective assessment of what is actually happening, right from the start. The 'start' of the incident can be a flexible concept. It may commence very suddenly with an unheralded flare-up of challenging behaviour. A member of staff may enter a situation already in progress, literally by entering the room where it is occurring. On the other hand there may be a long, slow build-up, with visible antecedents and triggers. However, whatever the nature of the 'start', that is the time to start assessing. It is a good working fundamental not to start doing anything until one has information about what one is doing something about. There are very, very few incidents where the terribleness of what is taking place is so extreme that there are not one or two seconds for a cool appraisal of how to pitch yourself into it.

Once again, this issue is fundamentally related to members of staff having the ability to remain calm and ordered. It is much much more difficult to assess a situation objectively if thoughts and feelings are racing, and more so if what is taking place immediately makes one frustrated and angry. This principle is also related to preparedness. The person who expects and accepts incidents of challenging behaviour is more likely to have the ability to assess the nature of the incident before acting.

Principle 7: 'tune-in' and stay sensitive to the other person's level of arousal

This is an aspect of assessment that is so crucial that it warrants the status of a principle of its own. Two key words appear in the title of the principle: 'tune' and 'sensitive'. Both of these things are aspects of good communication with anybody at any time. A good incident manager is a person who is being a good communicator during the incident. When communicating with another person at any time, nearly every person has the ability to 'tune-in' sensitively to all possible communications from the other. In particular, we look for the visual signals that accompany speech. Most human beings seem to have an amazingly refined ability to look, especially at the other person's face and body language, for the slightest, minutest changes in facial expression or quality of the eyes, which can give information about what that person is thinking or feeling at that moment. That information is then used to modify how the next statement to that person is phrased or what tone of voice used. It is easy to demonstrate this to oneself by observing two people in conversation for a minute or two.

Proper use of this ability is crucial to assess whether one is being effective in managing the incident; is everything cooling down or is the person becoming more aroused? Some of the things that can get in the way of tuning-in have already been discussed: it is difficult to tune-in when you are frustrated and angry, when you can't overcome the attitude that the person is in the wrong and the expectation that she/he should not be behaving like this.

Principle 8: maintain control of your own communication style and physical presence

The inner processes associated with this principle have been discussed. Naturally, they are about remaining calm, reflecting frequently on one's own emotional state during the incident, assessing and attempting to be a good communicator. There is more to it of course. Some advice on the 'nuts and bolts' of this is given in Chapter 9. The chapters by the contributors to this book contain many hints and tips on these matters. Chapter 9 reflects their contributions and is concerned with some detail on the very basic things like 'Where shall I stand or sit and why, what should I look like, how should I move, what shall I say, when shall I say it, how do I decide about all these things?'

As with the discussion of 'tuning-in' what it may entail is some seemingly awkward conscious thought about the things people do that are not normally given much conscious thought – facial expressions, tone of voice, movements, body language. We all use these things every instant of every day, we just tend not to think about them consciously.

Once again, the reality has to be faced that some people seem to be naturally very good at these things in challenging situations, or indeed all situations. Even more annoyingly, they may be so 'good' with their use of themselves, that they do not actually seem to have many incidents of challenging behaviour in their presence. They can often seem like people who are 'charismatic', or quietly powerful, or marvellously empathic. They may well have these characteristics, but the reality is probably that they are good communicators who have a powerful ability with physical presence and personal style.

During an incident of challenging behaviour a member of staff should be attempting to produce behaviour which is controlled and measured, not produced without a reason. This is a very high-order aspiration and it is indeed unlikely that any of us could achieve it. It is the striving for it as a principle of practice that is the important issue. Viewing its achievement as the objective, while accepting that perfection is not possible, is a realistic stance for a member of staff attempting to manage incidents of challenging behaviour effectively.

Principle 9: have prepared mental structures for helping you think and act

It is a good thing during an incident to have a framework or structure which can guide thinking and decision making or, better still, to have several to select from or which can influence each other. The best scenario is to avoid being left thinking 'What on earth shall I do next?' Some examples of such structures or frameworks would be:

- The list of principles outlined in this chapter. As already described, many staff are able to work creatively moment by moment, with their decision making and thinking underpinned by a set of principles which they consider to be valuable and right. A list of principles should not be so long that it is difficult to remember. On the other hand it should be long and detailed enough to provide a rich reference point for advice.
- A reasonably detailed verbal or written procedure, arrived at by evaluation and reflection upon previous similar incidents. This known procedure will also best be based upon values and principles of practice and be aimed at being effective for most staff most of the time.
- A contrived thinking and decision-making structure such as the 'stages of an incident ' (see Chapter 9). Such tools should again be brief enough to be carried in the memory, but detailed and flexible enough to provide some sort of answer when it is required.

Principle 10: use time effectively and creatively

One of the greatest stresses for staff is the time taken up with dealing with people's behaviour. This can lead to all sorts of feelings of failure, such as not giving appropriate time to people who are behaving well, not getting on with timetabled activities or the curriculum, feeling like a reactor to emergencies rather than the creator of positive experiences, feeling like there is no order in your classroom, workroom or house. I am always tempted to suggest that this stress is particularly heavy for teachers with the apparent general drive in education to get on with the curriculum and have observable pupil attainments at every moment. However, it seems that the stresses are not dissimilar for staff in other services. All services these days tend to have a powerful, understandable and (let's remember) in principle, totally laudable drive for the service-users to have continuous visible new attainments.

This stress can be one of the things which can lead staff into routine practices associated with attempting to quell and overpower the service user's behaviour – clamp tight external controls on it. Some people may have such forceful personalities that they may actually be quite good at it. These may often be the colleagues who make statements such as 'Well he doesn't do that in my presence'.

Finding a short-cut to managing people's behaviour that takes up less valuable time is desired by nearly all members of staff I meet. Unfortunately I don't really know one. The drawbacks to the clamp and control approach are various, and ultimately this style is one that cannot be recommended on many grounds. However, it is worth remembering that imposing external controls is actually one of the aspects of the style of practice recommended in this book. All of the contributors are attempting to help the service-users to be controlled, but it is not the only aspect of what they are doing.

The contributors do give advice on dealing with incidents of challenging behaviour as quickly as possible. The best route is for the staff and the service-user to become accustomed to the routine and the process involved, giving it the time it takes, and doing it well. This may result in incidents taking up less time by being dealt with more deftly. There is an attitude for staff, already mentioned, to accompany this orientation. The person's behaviour *is* the curriculum or work plan, not something that gets in the way of it. It is acknowledged that the way services are often constituted does not seem to reflect this outlook. Again, teachers may particularly make comments like, 'Well, tell that to the OFSTED inspectors'. Staff can feel that it is their job *not* to have challenging behaviours from their service-users and that they are supposed to be doing things quickly to overcome these behaviours so that other attainments can be made. A failure to get on with things feels like a failure in the eyes of the service.

I can only echo the frustrations when I feel that the staff I meet are indeed under these sorts of pressures, which are perhaps one of the reasons why it is necessary to have the more 'end-of-the-line' establishments such as those of Martin Bertulis and staff, and Bernie Hunt and staff. The service-users they work with have gravitated to them through other establishments. For the staff in Womaston and Oaklands College, Harperbury, there is no doubting the need to attend to the feelings and behaviour of the people they work with. That is what the staff are there for, first and foremost. However, perhaps some of the people they are working with would not have gravitated to their establishments were it not for some of the pressures described earlier in other services.

Principle 11: use teamwork

There are many aspects of teamworking which impinge on the effectiveness of practice during challenging situations. Virtually everyone acknowledges this, yet truly good teamwork can be a difficult thing to achieve. It is one of those areas where all of our personal human frailties are likely to become barriers to achieving communal human strength. The practical principles of good teamwork are straightforward, the emotional complexities of it can be anything but. Attempting to give detailed advice on resolving the personal and emotional obstacles to teamwork is not one of the aims of this book, indeed it would need another whole book to attempt this. However, there are many allusions to these issues throughout, and the contributors make suggestions about models of good teamwork and the strength they can draw from it.

This section briefly outlines features of teamwork which apply to staff working together during a challenging situation. Advice is offered here in statements which may well invoke the broader issues of staff relationships and further work at times other than during incidents, as with the first item:

- Don't be standing in the midst of an incident wondering what your colleague thinks about what you are doing. It is better to have certain knowledge by having had prior discussions as to technique, attitudes, values, ethos and working practices.
- Work is necessary also to achieve a situation where one member of staff does not step in abruptly and take over from another simply because they are more senior, more experienced, bigger, a man or a more powerful personality. Stepping in and taking over should be a matter of careful judgement.
- For regularly recurring incidents that are similar, have in place discussed and agreed procedures which are inline with values and accepted working practices.
- Maintain communication whenever possible with colleagues during incidents, either verbally or by exchanging looks and facial expressions.
- A normal good standard procedure is for only one member of staff to deal with the person exhibiting challenging behaviour. Other members of staff may well be there for support, but generally they should not talk to the service-user, and should give sensitive regard to things like: proximity – available, but not standing too close to the incident; body language, relaxed but available; and awareness, also giving proper attention to other things which may be happening in the room.
- Members of staff supporting another member of staff should 'tune-in' and read their colleague's emotional state as well as that of the service-user. They should be prepared to advise or to take over if one's colleague has clearly had enough.
- Members of staff relaying each other during long incidents is good standard procedure.

Principle 12: don't expect to manage all incidents successfully

This principle is a rather obvious one really isn't it? People are complicated, so are their feelings and behaviours. With the best endeavours in the world it is simply an unrealistic expectation that staff who work with people with learning difficulties are so well equipped with technique that they will handle all incidents successfully. It is surely better to accept this as a principle of practice. It not only helps enormously with the negative feelings associated with apparent failure, but also helps to generate positive feelings. These can include recognising the worth of an intervention (even if it wasn't perfect), having better attitudes toward evaluating positively and learning from the evaluation, and going home feeling okay even if there were several 'failures' during the day.

Additionally, staff have good and bad days. The bad days can arise for many human reasons and sometimes on those days one's practice will not be at the optimum. Working with people's challenging behaviour can be something of a daily grind. Success and effectiveness with a person needs to be monitored over a period of time, not just as a daily ritual of self-blame for not having 'won' that day.

Accepting 'failure' is part of a structure of positivity. This attitude can surely be seen in the work described by Bernie Hunt, Martin Bertulis, Maggie Roberts and Ann Vine. Staff who have the attitude that it will happen are usually in a better position to move forward, try different interventions, and to think creatively and imaginatively.

Chapter 6

Working with people with challenging behaviour in a further education class within a long-stay hospital

Bernie Hunt and Peter Brooks

Background

We work for Oaklands College of Further Education at the college annexe on the campus of Horizon Trust, Harperbury, a long-stay hospital for people with learning disabilities, near St Albans in Hertfordshire.

We work with two different groups morning and afternoon, in a session called 'Building Up To Independence'. We do try to make people as independent as possible, and a major aspect is to make people feel valued, and get them more settled in their behaviour, relationships and outlook. In that sense what we do is about independence. The afternoon group is more classroom-based with one community trip a week. The students' needs are in general more fundamental than the morning group where the focus is on getting out and about a little more.

Mostly our students are enrolled by ward staff. They are recommended and we go and visit them to see if they are suitable, whether they will fit in to the group we've got and what we as a team can do for them. Our referrals are almost always people with the most severely challenging behaviours – and the more challenging the better. Other day facilities here might have difficulty offering them anything and we feel that we're good at our job, we like working with the most difficult people. These are mostly people that have come from other institutions or who haven't been able to go into the community because of their challenging behaviours. All of the group at present are people who are living in the hospital, some on sections under the mental health act.

The building we work in is an old ward that we assume was a TB ward later converted to a day centre or some sort of nursing school, becoming the hospital school in 1971. In some senses it's an old and ramshackle building, but actually it's looking better than it has ever looked – it has been redecorated well and the classrooms are much more comfortable than at any previous time. It is one of the most ideal places for what we do there: all the classes are separated and you've also got a corridor – it is like a school or college. It can give people time out if they don't want to be in the room with you. We've got a super garden where people can just go and let off steam if they want to. We've got a corridor if they want to sit out or if they want to opt out. It's the perfect building, in all these ways but also because we've got used to our way of working in it. Our classrooms are really big so you can have two sides, with something going on one side and people who just want to sit and listen to music on the other side. That sense of big, available space is important. There are doors you can put across the middle of the room to protect people if a big incident occurs.

The students

It could be said that we are sort of an 'end-of-the-line' place. Most of our students have been in and out of all sorts of different provision and eventually ended up here because of their behaviour. The afternoon group is entirely composed of men, and they are all large. The average age in the group is about 30 and the students are all 6 feet or over. Because of their size, there are a lot of staff – smaller men and women – who naturally find them very intimidating straight away. Some typical descriptions follow.

Chris was a long-stay patient at another hospital. He was resettled for a short time in the community but his behaviour got worse. Very often the staff who are employed in homes have very little training, preparation or support. The staff may include two or three people that have nursing backgrounds and they will be in charge, but most staff are unqualified day care assistants who are given some training on-site. They are totally unprepared for the situations they come across. Usually it is then the people living in the homes who suffer and they are put back into institutions. Quite often we get the rejects, the people who come in very disturbed and up-tight about being moved around and about being treated badly – these people end up in our group.

Stephen has been in the hospital a long time and has had a resettlement but he too was not considered suitable there. He goes through phases of ripping his own and other people's clothes up. He gets quite up-tight if somebody's got something new. He doesn't tolerate any sort of loud noises or any bald aggression from people in our group and that will trigger him into ripping his clothes off. There is a look in his face that tells you he's going to do it – his whole face changes completely. He also had a fight with his mum the last time she visited – he actually ended up beating his mum up!

Ian can have very, very challenging behaviours. He bit part of Stephen's nose off because Stephen has always got his face in other people's business. Ian is a guy who's quite meticulous – he likes things tidy around him. He's also obsessive about washing up – he could wash up all the time. We try to help him with his obsession naturally, but we don't complain every time. He gets really anxious when Stephen starts getting up-tight. Stephen will rip tongues out of shoes – if someone has got a new pair of trainers Stephen will rip the tongue out and nothing's going to stop him. Ian is a runner – he can run 20 miles a day, literally non-stop.

All of them have good spells when you can actually get a lot going with them. Generally when they do present their challenging behaviours it's because they are misunderstood, or their communication skills aren't working and they're having problems with us. We haven't experienced a really big incident for over a year and a half, which is amazing because looking back on their records they've had really difficult times.

Personal background

Bernie

In 1984, when this was the old hospital school, I worked with people with profound and complex learning disabilities and challenging behaviours, and the approach then was entirely different – they were square pegs to be fitted into round holes. I felt uncomfortable with the approach, which was a classroom of maybe 10 or 11 students with task work. The student would have to sit down and do three tasks and they would get a mark to say whether they had done it or not, whether they needed prompting etc. Most students had done these tasks for years and they were asked to do them again and again and again. They were working how we wanted rather than with us working alongside and trying to understand them.

Then I left and had a baby and a break and thought I probably wouldn't ever go back. I did though, because when I started supply work I found that things had changed drastically. The staff working here by then were doing different things and trying out new approaches, particularly on communication. I found I wanted to come back and be part of it, and it's the best working-life experience I've ever had. To see those approaches work on students is the most exhilarating part of the job. You just know that the students are going to benefit. You can see these people just so stuck in a rut, and then they come in and you start working with them. You start helping the ward staff work that way with them and the changes are just incredible.

Some time after the school changed to further education officially, I became a lecturer, taking various types of classes. Then I was offered this job. I really wanted to do it because I like working with the people with the most difficulties. The job didn't have a good reputation, however, my colleague who preceded me in here had a bad time and got pretty badly beaten-up once.

Naturally, I get so much out of doing this job. One of the main things I think is the privilege of the students letting you in on their life. They can be so closed down, so insular, when they come in and they're so frightened. Suddenly this whole personality starts to unravel in front of you with just the first glimmers of a smile or the first fleeting eye contact, the first physical contact. All those things that they might have denied so many other people and they give you the privilege of having that with them – it's special. It's also very intellectually exciting, every day you have to think and think.

Peter

My title is Student Support Assistant. I wasn't a very good pupil at school, I didn't get good exam marks and my mother helped me towards this field of work. I started in an elderly person's day centre, where she worked, and stayed there for about three months. I built up relationships with certain older people that were absolutely fantastic – very good, life-affecting experiences – and it progressed from there. My mother left and went to Harperbury and I also did some supply work there, although for the first six months I felt absolutely useless. It was a completely different world for me and I found the first months very difficult. The whole Harperbury site was like a distant planet because it was so insular, so apart from everywhere else. A lot of the people there didn't realise what was going on in the outside world. I suppose I eventually found my place through being taught Interaction by Bernie. Eventually I did fit in and I was praised for my work after being here a while. I've been working here in the centre for five years now. It is very difficult to explain the job because in some weird sort of way I don't know really how I do it, but it's intuition, almost like a spiritual thing that comes out from inside. I feel like this job found me and I found it.

I started off with a group with various challenging behaviours in which Intensive Interaction was used much more. In that first group there were a lot of blind people, deaf people and people with profound and multiple learning difficulties, and we all shared a really good experience. I was with this group for about three years. Eventually I was moved along to work with another group – the 'Learning for Life' group – before coming to work with the group I'm with now.

How we work

The emphasis is on communicating and relating. Each student has an individual learning curve, and the most important thing for the majority of that group is to develop communication – with their own systems as the starting point. We work very hard to get the students more comfortable with relating to us and each other – this is a very basic priority. We also work hard to appreciate the way that they communicate and try to develop it. If they are going to be moving from the hospital this is the most important thing we can pass on to the staff who receive them. We can probably be more relaxed about this work than staff in the other facilities the students have been in and give it the time it takes – because the students have finally come to us.

We actually learn sometimes in the strangest way – when someone throws a cup of tea in your face you finally realise it's because they haven't got any sugar in their tea! So then we realise we must teach them the sign for sugar! But also just recording that information is one of the most important factors. For other staff to move on somewhere else with the person they need to know that the person does or doesn't take sugar, or what they hate, and so on. Likes and dislikes are one of the most important criteria when the students first join us. We generally have someone in the room for about six weeks before we do an initial assessment of their needs.

We do an assessment period for ourselves – we observe the person for six weeks or so. We don't expect anything too much from anyone within those six weeks, we just let them lead us, and we observe and take notes. After that I would do an initial assessment. We do a brief outline on social skills and general things about them and what their communication is like. We then have to work from where they are, which is the best way for us and them. After the first 12 weeks, we do an evaluation from the record keeping and use that evaluation to build up strategies. We make decisions about the way we will take that person, what they think they will benefit from and what we feel would be the best approach, and we work as a team on that. We would then work with that strategy for the next 12 weeks of term and then do another evaluation to see whether our stategy was working and whether the person achieved their learning goals within that time.

Working within further education requires that we work within certain structures of terms and courses and set learning goals. The criteria of a learning goal that we set and they are supposed to achieve can be difficult. We have to work with learning goals and set them, but we try to combine that with work on the old idea of the student's personal curriculum. That's the starting point for developing our aims and what we're working for. The main art is to think about sensible goals that are achievable. Setting them wrongly implies yet more failure for staff and students.

We still do individual evaluations each day. If a challenging situation happens then we will evaluate and think up strategies for dealing with that – what the trigger was, how we could defuse the situation, and how we feel about it. Then we're prepared the next time that situation happens. This steady process helps the students become much more trusting in you. You listen, you observe, you watch, you know, and they know that you know. Our students are not stupid – they've had years of observing people, they know who cares and who doesn't, and so once they know and trust you, they are very eager to perform. They trust you to handle their behaviour – they feel safe. They know that we understand why it's happening and after a situation you always say, 'Okay, we've done something wrong. Something's happened that's upset you. I know'. It is very important to reassure someone that you know that they're upset, and that you're not going to say 'Why are you doing this?' If you let them know that you understand they're upset that immediately acts as a calming strategy. Sometimes people are too upset to even hear what you're saying. We try to keep reassuring them. We know we haven't got all the answers.

Discussion between Bernie Hunt and the editor

What do you say to people who have the view that people you're working with should be dealt with very firmly, they need to controlled and if necessary punished for their behaviour, they've got to understand that their behaviour is not acceptable?

Initially you can't really talk to staff who are like that. You have to slowly re-educate them and you do that by working out a plan with that student and then letting others see it working and you hope that they'll work in that way. You can't suddenly tell someone who's qualified at their job that that's the route that they should be taking.

I was talking to someone recently who thought that one woman resident needed a 'tougher' approach and also perhaps needed behaviour modification programmes for certain behaviours. I tried to explain all the reasons why I thought she didn't need that done. The easiest way to explain it was to say we need to look more to the positive aspects of this person's life and less to the negatives, build-up the positives. One of the problems we can make for ourselves is to keep looking at the negative sides of the person's behaviour and give that a lot of attention. With all the students we work with, the negative sides of their behaviour will have had plenty of attention in the past. That purely negative side can become the person, not all of the positives. We find we don't have to sort of control and dominate the negatives, because we know we will get there by promoting the positives and coping with the negatives. You can't use punishment with anyone really. What you can do is build in boundaries once you get to know somebody.

How do you enforce the boundaries?

Through mutual respect.

How do you create that?

By building up relationships with people. Until you've got the relationship you can't have respect. They will respect you once that person has built up some trust in you.

I meet quite a few staff who use the term 'what this person needs is boundaries', and sometimes I sense that what they mean by that is that this person needs to be dominated and controlled.

No, I think it's something we'd work out between us. As the relationship establishes I could say to my student, 'No, you can't do that today, and if that's the way you want to go, is it really worth you coming here?' I might speak that way once I get to know somebody. Of course they want to come, they've built up a nice relationship, they enjoy coming and that's when you can start to build in some boundaries. It's not dominating somebody, it's helping them to fit in to the securities, to make them more sociable. It's very complex and it has to be done carefully and it can be done better once you've established a relationship and that person trusts you. You can link it into other environments then such as the ward, but it would have to be with somebody that knew them well, a key worker.

Naturally, we frequently end up preventing people from doing all sorts of things that they want to do. But that's different from giving them a set of rules to remember and live up to with their own self-control. What we're looking for is to help people to take some control of their lives and in order to do that they have to have some boundaries, but the boundaries are built-in to a whole relationship, they're not an abstract set of rules that you impose on them from the start. The necessary use of boundaries is of course an aspect of the way that we work, but it is not a definition of it.

So, from what you've told me so far, it seems to me that there is considerable space in the way that you work with your students for their behaviour and for them to have outbursts. Why don't you deal with them by immediately letting them know that those outbursts are unacceptable.

Because I don't know why they're having those outbursts, I have to experience those outbursts to find out what they're about. I can't easily stop them happening – that's part of my job – 'challenging behaviours'. It's my job for them to have those challenging behaviours with me so that I can experience them and work through them with the student. Having said that, we mostly now have a good system in the service where we get considerable information about a new student at the time of referral.

Isn't it your job to stop them having outbursts?

No, it's my job to find out why they're having them and to work with them on finding ways to reduce the challenges that they have. Quite often once they know that you know why they're having them, that's what stops them. Once you understand them then its all down to communication. It's them wanting to express something that they can't, something that's probably been bugging them for years. When you find out what it is, although you're not always right – it can take up to a year to find out – but you keep looking for routes in and the key to what it is that is upsetting them and what we can do to change, whether it's environment, or it could be a pair of trousers – it could be something that simple. They can't tell you, all they can do is express it in sometimes quite an aggressive way. I'd say too that of course we do help people to have less of their outbursts, but we don't achieve it simply by telling them not to have them.

Would you say you're successful with most of the people you work with?

There are some people who have been so badly traumatised in their life that they're not willing to accept anyone or a relationship with anyone. They're so shut down, so sceptical of people that they would rather withdraw and stay where they are – they feel safe. There are some exceptions and unless you work with them for 20 years you're never going to make any headway. For instance, there was one person who had been so sexually and physically abused that he was too withdrawn and shut down for us to help him with it in the time available.

How do you deal with the people who might come into the room after four weeks and say you still haven't got this person doing anything, it's your job to get this person doing things?

I would show them my record keeping, because every day I would be making observations on that person and writing them down. They might appear that they're not doing anything but they actually are – they're watching what's going on. You're looking for some eye contact during that session, even if it's just while making a cup of tea. There's little bits and pieces going on and as long as it's recorded, just attending is enough, just being in the room and being there is enough and tolerating a situation is enough. So, after about six weeks then, if they're not joining in or taking part in anything then I'd start thinking we've got to move on a bit with this person. So they would be allocated a one-to-one session with a member of staff each day, even if it's just two minutes or five minutes, whatever, they will have started building up a relationship. It might just be eye contact, or some facial regard, or just close proximity. It's just being with somebody. Even if a member of staff was just sitting with that person and commenting on what's going on in the room. Showing an interest in that person, making them feel valuable, a valuable part of the group.

It could sound like you're letting them do what they want, letting them get away with things?

Yes, I'm letting them do what they want but do they want to be there? They're brought to me, brought into a room and suddenly they have to sit there and watch what we're all doing and so they're not exactly doing what they want. They're, if you like, in a controlled environment. They're not doing what they want. They're there to learn and they are learning, they are learning some very basic skills that we have and take for granted.

You said that some of the people in that group are sectioned under the mental health act so I assume it's not unusual for you have new people coming in, it happens with reasonable regularity?

Yes. We might have someone coming in just on assessment. One was only with us for six weeks. After that six weeks he came to see us and bought us both a Snicker bar on the day he left. That was quite nice. He really chilled out with us. He was really sceptical when he came in. He had a lot of problems at home, he had tried to kill his mother and he wanted to move back near home but he couldn't live at home again. He was very frightened by his behaviour – he was very frightened about what he'd done. All the emotions he had about what was going on in his life, that was how they came out and he ended up with us. He really responded and we built up a super relationship. I had two chaps working in the class then, Peter and Andy. Andy is quite small and very quietly spoken and Peter's the gentle giant. They're two very cool people and really responsive to that age group and they knew exactly at what pitch and what level to go in at and it was just brilliant. He loved coming, he just wanted to be with them and be one of the lads. We built up a really strong relationship with him in six weeks and it felt brilliant.

You work very personally with the students. You work carefully with the things they are carrying around inside them which may be contributing to the way they behave. What are the 'personal factors' you find yourself working on most usually?

Helping them to find or bring out all the more positive aspects of their personalities and characters. That takes time, a sense of relaxed use of time and experience and confidence that you can do it. Sense of humour is a big one. Developing somebody's sense of humour is quite a breakthrough. It's one you've got to be careful with but it's one that's worth trying straight off, I think. The sense of humour is brilliant – if they know that you can have a laugh and they can too. It's wonderful when you see someone crack up laughing and then you can both laugh together about something. That's a really nice, warm feeling to share with somebody. So personality and character and sense of humour, I think.

I think also they may actually come in here prejudiced against staff – they've been through the system and hated it. They've trusted people and they've gone out of their lives. We're probably no better in their eyes than anyone else so you have to work really, really hard in reassuring them that you are consistent, you are there for them, you are there to help them, this is your job, I'm here, I'm here for you. That's worth telling people, that's worth saying, 'I'm here for you'. I doubt many people get told that. It's amazing that once somebody has jumped the hurdle and made the relationships, suddenly all the negative things aren't as important in their life as they were. I think self esteem is probably one of the most important things, building somebody's confidence up about themselves, just greeting them, being pleased to see them when they arrived.

But that's normal isn't it, being pleased to see one of the students?

When you see someone who's 6 feet 6 inches, walking down the corridor looking wild in the eye, you've still got to walk up to that person and greet them, saying 'Hi, how are you, you're looking good. I like your clothes.' That may be an experience this person doesn't get that often, given his size and his reputation. You've got to reassure them. Once they're inside the classroom you let them know. If I've got somebody new in I would let them find their own space. I'd greet them, they'd come into the classroom, I'd chat to them about what we do in the room. Whether they want to take part in that is up to them, but they could watch what we do. We'd be watching them as much as they'd be watching us – it's a two-way thing. I know that as much as we need to watch, so do they. That's part of our job, observation and they've been doing it for years. They're sussing us out as much as we are them. I find that works – for somebody to come in and actually be left alone and just watch what we're doing. Asking 'Would you like a drink? No? Well we're having a drink, would you like to join us for this?' Just the odd comment works. We're not going to push them into anything and if that goes on for six weeks, that's fine.

You work intensely on communication don't you?

That's the most important thing. That is the key. Once you can build up some sort of communication system and you are showing them that you are taking their communication system seriously – that you have recorded everything they do. Martin likes to use two knocks on the table as 'yes please', one for 'no'. If you ask him if he'd like a like a cup of tea or coffee that's what he'll do and unless you understand that you've got no idea of what he's doing. All their communication systems are recorded and that's a long process, that takes a long, long time to build up and for people to remember as well.

It's a central aspect of our staff style that we are responsive. The main theme of each session is that every student gets maximum opportunity for positive social exchanges with staff and other students. We concentrate ourselves on that, communicating with them about things and with a style that is meaningful for each individual. That's what we're about. Being communicative in that way links in with self-esteem issues and relating positively with other people. The more we get that going with each student, the less they are liable to be challenging. That positivity from us is just there. They don't have to do anything to earn it, you know, 'Behave well or we won't be nice to you'. It's there, it's always there.

It sounds like you do a lot of paperwork.

Yes, you do. You do a lot of daily recording. I used to keep it all but what I do now is an evaluation at the end of each six weeks and I have it all typed up and put on disk so when I come to do their end-of-year report I can have it all off the disk in one lot and I write the report from all their achievements over the year, and mine! There is a lot of paperwork for people with learning disabilities, but there has to be – it's the only way we can move on with them.

What about recordings on challenging incidents.

I keep behaviour charts, there's about four different sections in it – what the person was doing before, the environment, what triggered it, what was going on around the person when it happened. That's filled in and then filed with their paperwork and dated and timed.

So that gives you interpretations and statistics, so you've got full statistical records of the number of incidents during a given period of time. So six months later you know whether you're doing better, statistically.

The other thing that is recorded every day about a student is their well-being and that is a really important factor to how they're actually doing. If that person isn't well, if they've come in and they've got a streaming cold, they're not going to perform. You can't expect anyone to perform when they're like that and they don't often get a say in whether they can stay in bed or whatever, they are just sent to the centre so what we have to do is just make them as comfortable as possible.

Do you record anything about their mood for everybody everyday? Whether they were happy?

Yes, mood is always put under their well-being for the day, whether they were happy. I am meant to write my record-keeping as a learning record but I have to keep records that are important to me, whether so-and-so was in a good mood, whether they had clothes on that they were happy in. Whether they've had a hair cut, anything. I always record what we've chatted about as well because snippets of conversation are quite important. Once conversation starts it does prompt memory and you do get odd little bits and pieces that come out that probably happened over the weekend. You can always ask a member of staff and you can use it again. Once you know from a member of staff that they did do something at the weekend, like going to St Albans market and doing some shopping, you can bring that up again and reinforce that memory for them, 'Oh, you had a lovely time, didn't you, when you went to the market in St Albans' and it might prompt some more conversation and stimulate them into wanting to chat. So chatting is certainly on the agenda in our group! We try to make every activity as communicative as possible. Even if they don't want to do the activity, it's not necessarily about the activity. If art is timetabled, it's not about whether they produce a wonderful drawing, it's about stimulating the conversation around the table. It's just a joint focus that's making conversation happen.

Do you do any written evaluations of incidents, from the point of view of 'What did we do that worked?'

Some time ago a new group was started, one morning a week, with people who were difficult to resettle. I think they didn't have anybody else that would take this group but I fancied the challenge anyway, it interested me. So everything was re-arranged so that myself and another member of staff could take them.

The first week I had them I was in a totally unsuitable room with Peter and Barry, a new member of staff who had come from somewhere else but who knew the group of people. That was a big mistake. We got the class into this room that was used for resettlement, where they teach them home skills, what they do in their new home. I had three women screaming their heads off because they hadn't met me before and six men who were doing everything that they would do. So we had one guy absconding out one door, a guy trying to break all the light fittings. It was a nightmare, I was at screaming point and I thought, 'Right, calm down. Do what you do'. So we cordoned off this door that the bloke was trying to get out of with chairs so that there was only a small gap for him to get through. We couldn't lock it, but we'd have time to get to him before he got out the door. I thought the best thing to do was to give him one-to-one straight off. I said to Peter and Barry, 'Right we'll do some Intensive Interaction and we'll try to calm some of these people down. We'll work on some imitation, see what the group makes of it.'

It actually did calm down. I started working with the guy who was trying to abscond first and asked Peter to work with the guy who was trying break the lights and electric kettle and everything. I found myself getting very annoyed with this new member of staff, because everything I did he said 'Oh no, he doesn't like it when you go near him like that!' or 'Don't get to close to him, he'll whack you.' I was getting more and more worked up and then he put the radio on full blast. We'd just got the whole room settled down and he decided to go and put the radio on so I asked him to turn it off. He was working with one person, but he obviously felt very responsible for the group because he knew them and his input was very important because of that. We'd had quite a lot of chats before we'd gone over and he'd given us an awful lot of information about the group but what I didn't do, and I should have done, was fill him in more on the way we work. Because he'd worked elsewhere, in a classroom setting, I thought that he may have worked similarly to us but he didn't. He worked totally differently to us.

I thought I'd ask Barry to go and make some drinks so he went off and while he was off Peter and I got some nice interactions going with people and the rest of the group were really interested in what was going on. To my shock and horror, Barry walked out with a load of cups of tea already made. Sugar in them, everything. Everything was done, it was just nine cups on a tray all sugared and everyone had a cup of tea.

We carried on with what we were doing and I asked Barry to work with a lady who had started a little puzzle and he sat down with her . I asked Barry to stay with her for at least ten minutes, or until the student makes the choice that he doesn't want you there. Then this other guy, who was watching me do some interaction, grabbed hold of my hand and Barry informed me that that meant that he would like another drink (this was about a good three-quarters of an hour later). So I asked him if he'd like to come with me and make some drinks. He came into the kitchen with me and there was a trolley in there so I brought tea, chocolate, squashes and an assortment of biscuits. I wheeled this trolley out with him, with the kettle on the trolley and asked everybody to come up individually to make a choice of what drink they would like. Barry sat at the back saying 'They've not done this before, they won't know what to do.' I said 'Can we give them the chance, and see if they do. Most of them can probably point and make a choice of what they want'. It was quite apparent that they hadn't had a lot of choice-making in their lives, that Barry's was the way things were.

After a while, it took a good ten minutes nearly with each person, they actually did make choices of what they wanted, either by pointing or by picking up what they wanted. So they all made a choice and they all settled down and it turned out to be a reasonable morning after it being absolute chaos when we first went in there.

So it was very, very important that I did a very good evaluation of that morning, that I evaluated every single situation. I didn't do an individual record-keeping for each one of the group, it was just too chaotic, I just filled in odd bits on a total evaluation of the session. It was really important for Barry, particularly, to read what had happened, why it had happened and what we needed to do to stop that happening in future.

What were the skills that he didn't have?

He bombarded people all the time. His voice was too big. He was meant to be working with one person but he was busy talking to another one. He wasn't concentrating on the person he was with. He wasn't making them feel valued and important, he was busy looking round the room all the time. I think he felt responsible for the group because he knew them and wanted to share his knowledge. That was fine except that he was sharing knowledge loudly and frequently and was a jittery person to have in your team. He was working with this lady who had a puzzle out and you could see her looking at Barry and he was busy looking around the room. They were a challenging group and he had probably always had to be on his toes with them, rushing around. I want to teach him how to value a moment in time with a person. That the person that he's working with is the most important thing. Yes, at least one person has to give some overall attention to what is happening in the room, but not in the way that Barry was doing it.

What I did do was split the group up into three, so that we were responsible for three each. I gave Barry the ladies, because they seemed to be stationary, they weren't too much on the move. There was one who was crying a lot and needed calming and there was another one who was watching what was going on, she was really interested in what was going on around the room. The other lady had been crying, had been upset, and that was the person I wanted him to work with straight away. Barry wasn't focusing on what he was doing with that person and she was very aware that he wasn't focusing. You could see her face, when Barry got up and was rushing off to do something else, she was bewildered by what was going on, why aren't you with me? He worked with us for a long time after that and he was good, he really got the hang of the way we work and is a good person to have around. He just needed to do a lot of calming on himself, but that took time.

What was nice too was to have a new group like that, people who were pre-verbal who hadn't had Intensive Interaction before. For the others, the rest that weren't being worked with at any moment, they were just intent on what we were doing. They were so taken back with us joining-in with people. And the curiosity, I'd forgotten that curiosity can be there. Stopping and seeing if you're going to stop, doing something else, changing a pattern.

What are the qualities that a good, effective, member of staff is going to have in that, to do that work? What do you want the person to have in terms of skill and ability?

We want him to be able to key in to what they're doing, really focus on what they're doing and how the other person is seeing them. We want them to use their bodies and their faces and really make that person feel 'this is for me'. I think that the skills we're looking for are to be able to focus on the person and to be able to see what they're good at. Usually it's what they've perfected themselves over the years and if you can key in on something like that that they're particularly good at, imitating someone just flicking a wire around.

If they're not going to bombard people?

They should be quiet, maybe just gain eye contact. Just let that person know that they're there. Some people don't want you to – you know straight away if somebody's not going to enjoy interaction, they might get agitated very quickly, but most people that are active are quite curious about that. With quieter people you might perform a much quieter imitation, a small hand movement, facial expression and people generally like it, they generally smile. You get something back fairly quickly when you do friendly imitation.

In more general terms, just being with the group, what are you looking for in a member of staff?

A calmness, a real calmness. I don't want someone who's going to shout across the room 'Oh, he's the one that will break the lights'. A member of staff needs to be a person who has a simple vested interest in people – all people. A willingness to learn, every moment is a learning situation. You need to be able to work through your own problems, I think working through your own emotional stuff happens to people in this work . . . flexible thinking, all the time . . . you've got to deal with your own need to blame people.

What about their personal deportment?

When somebody's new they're quite nervous and their body language is quite nervous as well. That makes me twitchy when I've got a group. It doesn't matter if the student's body language is nervous, I can deal with that, but with a member of staff it's quite difficult. So I really needed Barry on home ground to sort that out, with people that I was totally used to. He could have fitted into a group in my classroom fine and been shown the ropes, but a totally new situation with a completely new class and a completely new environment was really difficult.

Peter has developed this ability to mould himself to the situation. He's gentle and he's got this ability to make himself appear small, even though he's 6' 5". He makes people feel safe. Then he can also be very animated, using lots of facial expressions with a huge expanse of body language. When we are having fun he is larger than life, his animation in the room is massive and the students really respond to that. But when the chips are down he knows how to go gentle and slow. On the other hand, you can have a member of staff whose body language is really quite quiet and demure, but the students respond to that too. They've got this general aura of quiet and calm – steadiness. That's a nice body to have in the room as well.

How do you want a member of staff to use their voice, generally, not just in one-to-one?

101

Quietly and not say the obvious! It's very difficult, I can't think what it is that we all learn together but we do all learn something together. Quite often you think of something to say but you think, 'No, this isn't the right time to say it now, I'll say it after the session'. It doesn't help people to state the obvious. It doesn't help to say, 'Oh, if he goes out there, he'll do a wee in the corner'. One member of staff had recently had a baby and he was very much into the interaction and he learnt very quickly, he's bright and he picked up the stuff very quickly. He now runs the Thursday group at another hospital and he does really really well. He's using it to hopefully achieve his teaching qualification. He'd worked with me for two terms and he was just excellent at the job. He just had the right attitude from the start, he was compassionate.

What word would you use to describe the ethos and the atmosphere of your room?

I give people a sheet when they come in and it's got 'rules', I don't like people talking about personal things about the students, I don't like them talking in front of them. There's a whole list of things on it, if we're having conversations ourselves it's important that students are always included in conversations. It's our group.

How do you stay calm when the chips are down? What have you got going on in your head?

When things are absolutely hectic, I have to think 'This is what I'm about', this is when it's professional. I have to think 'This is why I do the job I'm doing' and I've got to stay in control. I've got to keep my assistants calm and I have to take the initiative, I have to be in control and I know all the key factors, I know how things work, I just have to put them in action, and that what's I do.

It always works? You never lose it?

Not yet. I have cried after a situation. I have to have debrief with all of us. It's not always completely spot-on, there's always room for improvement and you always have to talk that through and say next time we could do so-and-so, 'Okay we kept it all at an even keel and nothing too drastic happened', and if someone came up with a really good idea then let them know it was a good idea. They've used their initiative.

That's when you're debriefing on incident management?

Yes. It's about putting everything you've learned into practice at that moment in time. When everything blows up in the air you just have to. We were on the bus once, and it was an old, great big yellow bus, that we'd borrowed, like an ice-cream bus. We had an incident with a lady getting out of the seat and she'd taken all her clothes off on the bus in full view of some passers by. We'd had to pull over in this lane. As I'd got up I hadn't realised I'd caught my trousers or my cardigan on the handbrake and it had come off and here we were trying to deal with this lady who had stripped and was biting and the bus was rolling down the hill! You have to be on the ball.

So when you've got a new member of staff, what tips do you give them about keeping calm?

For new people it's best to observe in a situation, to let the people who've been there longer deal with a situation and for them to observe what's going on. As I would say to one of my students, 'Don't worry about feeling like you're not doing anything, the most important thing for you to do at the moment is observe. Just watch what we're doing, how we're talking, how we're acting. You just try and work in that way. It goes full circle, that is communication from student to staff, to student. But also, it's my job to protect new staff until they've got the hang of things. I think I didn't get that right for Barry that morning. Nothing terrible happened, but I didn't read him and protect him enough.

Have you ever shouted?

Peter would probably tell you whether I've shouted in a group or not. I don't think I have, I may have in a certain situation. I do shout at home, with my kids. They shout at me as well. It's probably counter-productive with them too, but it's harder not to do it.

You've almost got a rule about that?

Yes. And I think we all find it easier not to lose it because we've got each other, we've got a team and we always understand that someone else can step in, it's not a problem to do that. Plus, we spend a lot of time laughing – there's not much that can happen that we don't have a laugh about afterwards. Oh yes that's another staff quality, juvenile sense of humour.

But why not, loads of staff who do our work shout?

Yeah, well. Hmmm. Once, I was talking to a social worker in the staff room and I heard Cathy (a colleague) shouting, really yelling in the corridor, and I was so shocked I stopped talking and I stood up, I couldn't believe what I was hearing. I looked down the corridor and I turned to the social worker and said, 'Oh, it's okay, she's talking to her dog'. I've never heard anyone talk to a student at Harperbury like that, ever. Well, not for years and years, since the old days. The people that work here would not talk like that to anyone. I was so shocked I thought 'Cathy has lost it, she's totally lost it'. Anyway, she'd got her dog out of the car and he'd shat in the corridor. I was thinking, 'What the hell, so what if a student's done a poo in the corridor?' I was thinking what on earth is she doing . . . and it was her dog!

What are your rules for yourself about managing incidents of difficult behaviour?

Calm voice, try and keep it calm. I think you can tell people off, if you like, when it's diffused. That's when you can take a stronger tone and say, 'Look that really upset me and other people in the classroom. Why? Where did that come from? What was it about?' But when it's happening you have to stay really calm, you have to keep a really controlled voice. You have to let them know that if they're not in control you are, you're there and it's temporary, it's keeping it on an even keel for them, not letting it escalate into anything. You walk up and say, 'OK, come on calm down', you'll try and keep an even voice.

What's your voice like?

Very calm. Probably as I'm talking now. I say 'Look has something really upset you?' Maybe apologise for the other person – I'll say 'Look I'm really sorry this has happened – maybe that person didn't intend to do that to you'. It's a very soft approach. You need a calm voice.

Do you think about proximity? What sort of rules do you have on that?

It depends on the person. I have walked into a situation when I've not been well and I've not thought it through. I've walked straight into a situation and I've got really hurt, really whacked across the side of the neck.

I think it's good eye contact as well. Your voice and how you are. I approached somebody one day, quite a big man, who immediately smacked me on the knees. I took four paces back and bent down on the ground so I was actually on a low level. I had made myself a lot smaller – almost empowering him. I had just come over and for all he knew I could have been another student. I suppose I defused that situation by just being on the ground, moving away and keeping good eye contact. After a while he requested some pens and pencils. I still kept at that distance. Generally talking to him softly, giving him eye contact.

Some people say you have to be careful about eye contact?

It depends how you look at someone. If you look at someone with your eyes relaxed, your whole posture, your eyes, your mouth, everything has to be really relaxed. Trying to keep your voice on an even keel, reassuring them that it's okay, they can express these feelings if they want to as long as they don't hurt anyone else. If they want to leave the room they can, giving them ways out. Trying to see them through it, whatever it is they're trying to express and what they're experiencing. The worst thing you can say is 'What's the matter?' A lot of people with learning disabilities, before they blow, say 'What's the matter?' because that's what they're used to having said to them. With one of my students you know that that's when she's going to blow, so I know that it might be a good idea to take her out for walk or something.

And reading the person?

When you're doing your job you have to read their eyes, their body language. Whether they're lashing out, you just know how near you can get. Eventually you probably can put your arms around them and say, 'It's all right, you're OK'. Sometimes you do get it wrong, if you're feeling a bit vulnerable or a bit low you do just walk into a situation and you can get hurt then. You have to be very careful if you're feeling a bit low or a bit under the weather, and it's worth sharing that with your team so that they know if an incident happens they should take the lead and not you.

What you've got naturally, you've developed naturally and you find difficult to articulate, I have to try to teach that to people from the word 'go', maybe because they're people who shout a lot and get in people's faces and don't give proper regard for proximity and arousal levels, and they need to be taught it on a course or slowly by working with me and the others. Telling them to work like that is one thing, helping them to know how to do it is another.

Summarise: what would be some good tips on managing incidents of challenging behaviour?

- Staying calm.
- Think about where you put yourself.
- Use your voice well and eye contact.

Chapter 7

Developing practice in a residential team – training, talking, thinking, working

Tracey Culshaw and Karin Purvis

Introduction

In this chapter we describe our experiences and work with a group of adults with learning disabilities who present challenging behaviour. These people all live in a small purpose-built residential unit for people with challenging needs. We will look at our joint approach for working towards reducing incidents of challenging behaviour by promoting quality relationships and addressing the communication needs of our clients. These ways of enhancing people's lives and increasing their self-esteem and self-worth went hand in hand with supporting and developing the skills of the staff team who worked with this client group. Firstly, an introduction into who 'we' are:

- I am Tracey Culshaw (TC). I have worked with people with learning disabilities for over seventeen years in a variety of settings. I have worked in day centres, residential homes and colleges and have also worked in the United States and Romania. I first qualified in teaching people with learning disabilities (CFETMHP), but later went on to study counselling (Ad. Dip. in Cons). In the latter part of my work I have been more involved in working with people who not only have a learning disability, but whose behaviour is also deemed to be challenging. It is during my time working as a manager of a unit for people with learning disabilities and challenging needs that I first met Karin.
- I am Karin Purvis. I qualified as a speech and language therapist nine years ago. For the last eight years I have worked as a specialist speech and language therapist for people with learning disabilities. During this time, I have become more involved in working with people with challenging needs and the staff who support them.

We have worked together for almost five years. When looking at our clients' 'challenging needs' we have focused on their interaction with others and their communication needs.

Background information

The individuals we currently work with are all deemed to have 'behaviour which challenges the service'. The majority of them had previously lived in long-stay hospitals for people with learning disabilities, often more than one hospital. A few people had lived in community settings which had broken down. These people were difficult to place due to their behaviours. The behaviours displayed included hitting, kicking, biting, scratching, throwing objects, damaging property, smearing, inappropriate urination and spitting. The common factor linking each of these individuals was that they all displayed difficult behaviour.

The behaviours had been managed in many different ways, the majority being on a control and restraint basis, as this was seen as the most appropriate way, given the extremity of the behaviour being displayed. One of our major perceptions was that each person had very low self-esteem and difficulty in forming quality relationships and this was reflected in their behaviour. We believe these individuals would not have actively chosen to live together as a group.

None of the individuals had a detailed assessment of their communication skills by a speech and language therapist. Most had good expressive language, and were able to speak using complex sentences, although one person had no expressive language. Care staff judged the individuals to have good receptive language/verbal comprehension, and felt that they understood most of what was said to them. This led to misconceptions and individuals sometimes being labelled as, for example, stubborn, wanting to hurt people, etc.

Although there were records detailing the injuries sustained by staff and clients, and consequences of the behaviour (e.g. medication given), there was little information on the antecedents to the incidents.

A lot of information needed to develop future care plans to enable people to be supported was available by asking staff, some of whom had worked with the people for a number of years. Although this had advantages, there were also some disadvantages. Some of the information about how individuals could be supported was preconceived. Much of what was remembered involved incidents in which people were seriously injured, leading to clients developing reputations. This reputation was sometimes transmitted to the individuals themselves, often subconsciously through non-verbal information (e.g. body language, tone of voice, facial expression).

To support clients and staff more effectively, the following issues needed to be addressed:

- It was necessary to develop consistent ideologies and philosophies for a staff group from a mixed background on working with individuals whose behaviour could challenge.
- Methods of supporting staff in a potentially difficult working environment had to be established.
- Staff needed to be encouraged to look at the possible communicative function of the individual's behaviour.

- The development of the client's self-worth and self-esteem was fundamental.

Two elements underpinned these issues:

- the development of meaningful interactions/relationships;
- communication.

Methods for facilitating change

Relationships and interactions – Tracey Culshaw

Our picture of ourselves, our self-image, is built upon the way in which people interact with us, i.e. what they say and do. This can be on an individual, group or societal level. When I first started to work with the clients, I was very aware of the negative messages that they had received, directly and indirectly, on all these levels. The messages had generally been as a direct response (reaction) to an individual's behaviour/actions. This in itself created a circle of negative interactions, which led to the clients having low expectations of themselves and very poor self-image/self-esteem. One of the ways of changing this set pattern of behaviour was to encourage positive interactions and relationships, and this was one of my main aims for the unit.

To enable this to happen, staff needed to differentiate the person from their behaviour. Most staff–client interactions were based on what the person did (i.e. their behaviour), and not who they were. There was a sense that their identity had been lost, and that they had *become* their behaviour. Separating the person from their behaviour was essential to build up the caring, empathic relationships that were desired within the team. Once the person was viewed in this way, staff could then look more clearly at what the person was trying to communicate. This 'listening' went hand-in-hand with the Somerset Total Communication training that staff were receiving.

Furthermore, by not working within a punishment model, the 'power relationship' is eroded, resulting in the client feeling more equal and valued. Punishment prevents a client from doing something on the basis of us, as staff, saying 'No'. The power and control is in our hands. The client is dependent on us and cannot be self-determined and make a choice. The ability to empower a client when we are working with them is very important. Our clients often have to rely on us for many things. We, as staff, often make many of the decisions in their day-to-day lives. Staff have the power to make things happen or not happen. While I recognise this is inevitable in some circumstances, we need to constantly evaluate this and ensure that we are giving clients every possibility to take control (where they can) of their lives.

When working with our clients there are still several issues that we need to consider for each individual and discuss with the staff team. Some of these issues are:

1. How are we going to promote a person's self-respect, self-worth and self-image when they display behaviours which can be deemed to be challenging and/or socially inappropriate?
2. We need to understand the purpose and possible communicative function of the behaviour. Does it just reinforce what a person feels/thinks about themselves or how others feel/think about them? Is it the only way they know to communicate a feeling or thought?
3. We often have pictures or details about our clients that tell us how they communicate their likes and dislikes. These are often listed with other factual details in files, to build up a pen picture of the individual. We often do not have information about the way in which the person communicates how they *feel*. It is very difficult to judge whether someone is sad as opposed to bored, happy as opposed to content, angry as opposed to frustrated or in pain. How do we know how our clients are feeling? Do all staff have the same knowledge/views?
4. It is impossible to judge the communicative function of the behaviour if we do not know how the person communicates each feeling. Often the client is not aware of the differences and complexities of the different emotions. This in itself can be the reason for some behaviours. They may not know that they are feeling angered by a situation or person, but they may not like the physical sensations they are experiencing. This may be in the form of actual physical pain. Being frightened can cause stomach ache and being angry can cause headaches, etc.

Environments

When I first started working with this particular client group, their immediate living environment was sterile and impersonal. The reason cited for this was to protect the individual(s), so that they could not harm or injure themselves with the furniture. Therefore, the living room consisted of plastic-covered chairs, a television behind a plastic screen 6 feet up the wall, metal key-controlled light switches (only members of staff had a key to operate the lights), and a table fixed securely to the floor. There were no pictures, soft furnishings or anything to help promote a positive self-image for the individuals living there.

The first move was to give a strong non-verbal message of valuing a person by creating a homely atmosphere. This involved redecoration and replacing all the furniture with heavy-duty everyday chairs, tables, lamps, pictures etc. The television was moved to floor level and carpet was laid on the floor. Each person's bedroom was refurbished with furniture and colour schemes that were chosen by them. Each bedroom was very individual and reflected the personality of the individual it belonged to. Bedrooms were encouraged to be seen as safe places where people had personal space to work out their emotions. One client in particular has, on several occasions, thrown his personal effects around in his room when he has been unable to control some of his feelings. This was seen as a positive move, because he was not throwing things at other people or hitting out (i.e. putting them at risk), which were behaviours that he had previously displayed when emotions were high. This change in behaviour did not happen overnight. It required a great deal of hard work by both the client and staff, and was only possible because a secure relationship of trust had been established.

Training course: meeting a challenge

To help staff to understand the relationship between their interactions and the client's behaviour and the philosophy base I wanted them to work within, a one day course was devised. The course was named 'Meeting a challenge' and covered several areas i.e. definitions of challenging behaviour, vicious and learning circles, labelling, Maslow's Hierarchy of Needs (Maslow 1970), and the relationship between communication difficulties and challenging behaviour. The course also included a session on releasing techniques which enabled staff to work more safely and confidently with clients.

The first part of the course encouraged staff to look at their own 'problem' behaviours, e.g. what we all do when we are feeling angry, upset, sad or frustrated. A list was made of these behaviours, e.g. swearing, shouting, kicking doors, crying, bingeing, sulking, throwing things. Another list was made of our client's 'problem' behaviour and the two lists were compared. This highlighted the fact that we all display, at times, some of these 'challenging' behaviours. The main difference was in the frequency and/or duration of the behaviours. We acknowledged that our clients were likely to potentially experience more triggers, e.g. lack of freedom of movement or of privacy, and they may not have access to the coping strategies we use, e.g. getting drunk or being alone. There were other behaviours on the client list, e.g. smearing, self-injurious behaviour.

A discussion took place on people's views on why these other behaviours may occur. Staff pointed out that people who do not have a learning disability sometimes display these behaviours when they are very stressed. Most staff either knew or had read about someone trying to hurt themselves as a way of communicating how unhappy they were. Some of the behaviour was thought to be a reflection of the extent of the client's learning disability and/or their emotional development. One particular 35-year-old-man was documented as having an emotional developmental level similar to a three to four year old; he showed behavioural responses to situations that you would expect from a person whose emotional level was three to four years of age. The staff had not considered this link previously and, in the light of this knowledge, could re-evaluate the client's behaviour and how they viewed and supported the client.

Working closely with the Psychology Department, programmes could be devised to look at how to support this client. Staff stopped expecting the client to take control of his own behaviour and acknowledged that certain situations triggered an outburst of emotion. The challenge for staff was to try to prevent these triggers until more work could be done in helping the client to develop other strategies to express his feelings and for staff to defuse the situation and reassure him. This client does seem to have matured emotionally in the way he deals with certain situations, which I feel is a reflection of the success of a consistent joint approach by everyone.

The second part of the course went on to look at what affects people's behaviour, i.e. medication, attitudes, places, space, noise, people, activities, personal history, changes, abuse, feelings, mental health, physical health, communication and verbal comprehension to name but a few! This part of the course helped staff to have a greater understanding of a client's behaviour. This greater understanding meant that staff could more readily separate the person from their behaviour and build up a greater empathy with the client.

The section on communication and verbal comprehension was expanded by the speech and language therapist and is covered elsewhere in this article. This section had a very positive effect on staff as this was something they could change, whereas many of the other possible reasons for a client's behaviour could not be changed. Staff could only be aware and sensitive of, for example, a client's previous history. The role of the speech and language therapist was highlighted. Staff had the opportunity to look at the role they can play in helping a client to communicate how they feel, and look at the possible communicative function of a client's behaviour.

Communication – Karin Purvis

The relationship between communication and behaviour is well documented. Much research has focused on the fact that challenging behaviours are often associated with communication difficulties, and that challenging behaviour often has a communicative function. Our observations suggested that all of the clients had significant communication difficulties despite their apparent expressive language ability. To establish the level of communication difficulties, each person was referred for speech and language therapy assessment. Although individuals had very different communication skills, detailed assessment highlighted the following general points:

1. Receptive language and verbal comprehension was at a much lower level than expressive language. Difficulties in this area were masked by a reliance on situational understanding, familiar routines and non-verbal cues. The use of complex expressive language, particularly echoed and learnt language and good social conversation, also masked verbal comprehension difficulties. It is a human trait to 'hide' those characteristics which make us feel at a disadvantage, and clients had developed very effective strategies for masking their difficulties.
2. Everyone had specific difficulty in understanding emotions, negatives and time concepts. Most people had difficulty with social interactive skills, particularly respecting personal space, initiating conversations, turn-taking and understanding social rules.
3. There was enormous variability in communication skills within individuals, depending on other factors, such as health, mood, medication and environmental issues (e.g. noise, location, time of day/week).

In common with most speech and language therapists for adults with learning disabilities, I have a large caseload spread across a wide geographical area – the clients living in this particular unit formed a very small, but time-consuming part of my caseload. It has long been recognised that the onus for communication work should lie with care staff – the people who have day-to-day contact with clients, and that the speech and language therapist should act as a consultant (Cottam 1986, Calculator 1988).

As speech and language therapists may be doing less hands-on work with clients, there is a real danger that we will be seen by care staff and clients as being near-strangers who come into the Unit only occasionally and dispense advice with little regard for the practicalities of this advice being implemented by care staff. As we do not work in the unit regularly, we have little perception of how the unit functions and the demands placed on staff.

I spend approximately one-third of my time involved in staff training. I consider this to be time well spent for two reasons. Firstly, staff are given the opportunity to develop knowledge and skills which will enable them to communicate more effectively with clients – this is essential. Secondly, it provides an opportunity for me to meet staff and vice versa, and provides the foundation for us to build a working relationship.

It is preferable that clients have the opportunity to meet the speech and language therapist before any kind of assessment is attempted, although this is not always possible. I involve staff in the assessment of individual client's communication skills, because they have an enormous amount of knowledge about how their clients communicate in different situations. The presence of a familiar member of staff also reassures the client that everything is okay.

Staff are involved in planning communication programmes and monitoring their effectiveness. This is important – if staff are to implement advice on a day-to-day basis, the programmes need to be practical and relevant. Staff will have a valuable contribution to make should a programme need to be changed, because they will have a good idea of what has been successful or unsuccessful.

In addition, I feel very strongly that the speech and language therapist should, when appropriate, work with the client, e.g. I have, at times, taken the lead role in explaining a major change to a client using signs and symbols; this is then reinforced by staff in residential and day care. This has helped me to be more realistic and has done staff a power of good on the occasions when I have got it wrong!

An outline of my involvement in staff training and working with individual clients in this particular Unit, follows.

Staff training

Before any effective work with individual clients could be carried out, it was necessary to undertake staff training. Training needed to focus on the development of communication in people with learning disabilities, ways of developing communication skills and the relationship between communication and challenging behaviour. Staff attended training in the use of Somerset Total

Communication (STC) and more specific training on communication and challenging behaviour.

Somerset Total Communication

The Somerset Total Communication Project (STCP) was established in 1991. It is a county-wide scheme which comprises a needs-led vocabulary of signs and symbols, a comprehensive support network for care staff and a three-tier staff training structure. STCP is co-ordinated by the Speech and Language Therapy Service and is promoted and supported by the Social Services Department and the Health Service (Jones *et al.* 1992, Purvis 1996, STCP Resource Base).

All care staff in the Unit completed the basic induction level of the STCP training programme. This is a seven-hour course which covers the following:

- basic knowledge about the development of STC;
- reasons why STC is used;
- finger spelling;
- 100 signs (60 basic, 40 chosen by the Unit staff);
- basic symbols;
- key words and signing simple sentences.

Two staff also completed the 'top' level of training and were designated STC co-ordinators. Their role was to teach induction level STC to the staff team, implement and promote the use of STC within the unit, cascade information about STC to staff and to be a 'link' person between the speech and language therapist and the unit.

Co-ordinator training covered the following areas:

- approximately 400 signs, signing sentences and conversation;
- the development of communication skills in people with learning disabilities;
- selecting sign and symbol vocabularies and methods of teaching these to individual clients;
- generating signs and symbols;
- meeting staff objections to the use of STC;
- teaching Induction Level STC.

Meeting a challenge

I also taught on a section of the 'Meeting a challenge' course mentioned previously. This contribution was designed to be experiential. It looked at the relationship between communication and challenging behaviour, ways in which communication may break down, and basic ways of working with people with communication difficulties (e.g. general approaches and the use of symbols).

Staff requested that this section of the course should be more detailed. Consequently, a half day course entitled 'Communicating with your feet' was developed.

Communicating with your feet

This course covered the following:

1. the cyclical relationship between communication and challenging behaviour;
2. the value of communication and the relationship between communication and behaviour in all of us;
3. communication breakdown and alternative strategies used by clients;
4. the importance of establishing the possible communicative function of the behaviour, particularly if it concerns the health of the individual – the importance of multi-disciplinary input in establishing this, is emphasised;
5. the effect of life history and past experiences on communication;
6. introducing techniques which may help:
   (a) using symbols to develop concepts of emotions, time and negatives, etc.;
   (b) the importance of staff using appropriate non-verbal communication and interpreting the non-verbal communication of clients;
   (c) the importance of consistent communication strategies being used by *all* staff in *all* environments;
   (d) recognising differences in individual clients and being flexible in meeting these differences.

Working with individuals

I assess the individual's communication skills in collaboration with care staff and the multi-disciplinary team (particularly the clinical psychologist for people with learning disabilities). Communication programmes are then written and discussed with the unit manager. These are implemented by care staff. As care staff work with clients every day, it is more appropriate for them to be responsible for developing and maintaining a consistent and suitable communication environment that meets the needs of the individual and the group. This is monitored by the unit manager and myself, and additional support is given when required. It is important that staff are involved in developing communication programmes, because they need to feel comfortable in implementing the recommendation made.

It is impossible to identify one specific way of working, because of the highly varied nature of the communication skills of the individuals within the Unit. Outlines of some methods that have been found to be particularly useful with more than one person follow.

Adapting communication

Staff are encouraged to observe and be sensitive to the communication skills of individual clients, and to pass this information on to others. They have to be skilled at recognising people's idiosyncratic communication (e.g. gestures, body language, tone of voice) and be able to adapt their own communication to an appropriate level.

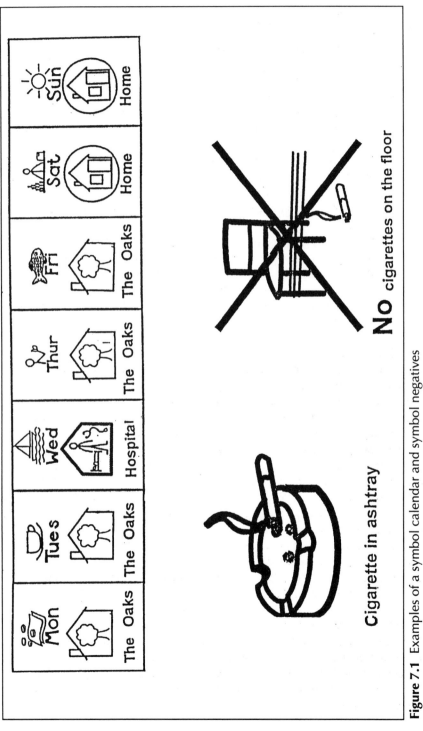

Figure 7.1 Examples of a symbol calendar and symbol negatives

Interaction skills

In addition to the work already outlined, it has been necessary to focus more specifically on the development of basic interaction with one client. This has been achieved using the Intensive Interaction approach. (Nind and Hewett 1994)

Time concepts

Some clients showed considerable anxiety over the timing of events. We worked hard to create identical symbol calendars in residential and day care. Every day, clients move an arrow on to the appropriate day and, over time, learn the sequence of the days of the week (see Figure 7.1). Symbol calendars can then be used to explain change and significant events. The complexity of calendars is adapted according to the needs of the individual e.g. one person has an appointment diary in symbols, another individual has a monthly or weekly calendar.

There was some difficulty with staff rotas, particularly with one person who became anxious if favoured staff members were not on the rota. We are presently working towards use of photographs of staff on a wallchart as a visual rota for clients.

Appointment diaries using symbols and clock stamps are also used. This has been a useful and functional way of teaching people to tell the time, and understand the sequence of time, with some clients using a personal symobl diary.

Negatives

We often may not give sufficient attention to the posibility that large number of adults with learning disabilities have difficulty in understanding negative structures. It is imperative in our work with people with difficult behaviour that we are able to use negatives effectively. It is very easy for the negative marker to become 'lost', particularly if the client has poor verbal comprehension e.g. 'We are not going swimming' sounds very similar to 'We are going swimming'. Contracted negatives, e.g. 'We aren't going swimming' are even harder. If a client understands only one key word, it is likely to be 'swimming'. Further confusion may arise if staff are using non-verbal cues associated with negatives (e.g. facial expression, tone of voice, shaking their head, etc.) but the client does not understand that a negative has been used verbally.

We found that all of the clients in the unit have difficulty in understanding negatives and we needed to focus more attention on this. We found no one preferred way of teaching this concept. Assessment has identified the way in which each individual can be supported to understand negatives. Methods can be quite diverse, depending on the person's communication levels and called for attention to what might be obvious details, but some of the methods below were particularly successful, for instance with one person who had poor etiquette with his cigarette ends:

1. Using visual reminders:
   (a) having lots of ashtrays around as a reminder to use them (easy to forget to provide them);

    (b) using symbols with red crosses through them (see example, Figure 7.1);

    (c) signing 'No' and clearly modelling appropriate body language (e.g. head shaking).

2. Using speech, signing and symbols in diverse ways to get the negative structure across. The method used will depend on the individual:

    (a) setting the subject first: 'Cigarettes on the floor – No';

    (b) Using the negative first 'No cigarettes on the floor';

Some people find this difficult to follow: they focus on the 'No' and 'miss' the rest of the sentence, so:

    (c) Giving a positive first: 'Put cigarettes in the ashtray. No cigarettes on the floor'.

It is important that the tone of voice and body language consistently indicate 'No', with firmness, but without being confrontational. The issue for staff is the cigarette on the floor, and not one of making the person needlessly feel bad. Once a successful way of presenting negatives has been established, it is essential that this method is used consistently everywhere and by everyone.

Record keeping and incident management – Tracey Culshaw

It was important to develop a system of accurate recording as incidents happened. There was no clear and consistent system in place, so it was difficult to find out factual information about an incident. There was no clear definition of what was and was not an incident. If a member of staff was hurt when working it was often only recorded that a bruise or injury had been sustained. Many 'incidents' were not recorded, because no injury had occurred. Most incidents were recorded on an accident form. This form was devised for recording accidents, and so had no space to record information concerning behaviour before, during and after the incident, and there was no room to record whether a care plan was used, and whether it had been successful. There was no accurate information on how often or why a client had been upset or angry, or whether staff had been able to successfully divert the behaviour. This information was essential in evaluating and monitoring the effectiveness of care plans.

I wanted to introduce a simple, uniform system which recorded *all* incidents, and whether care plans were used. This would mean that an accurate overall picture could be devised about any individual client over any given period of time. The incident form was devised to ask the questions I wanted answered. Accident forms still needed to be completed separately, but photocopies of these were attached to the incident form. This was to ensure that accident forms were completed. To prevent staff having to write things twice, the forms could be cross referenced. Each incident form had a reference number and they were all kept together in an Incident Folder rather than with individual client's case notes. A reference to the incident file could be written in the daily care notes. At the foot of the incident form was a space for the date and the signature of the person completing the form, and there was also space for the shift leader and myself to sign and date the form. At the front of the incident folder was a form where the date, reference number, client name, nature of incident and space for the line manager to sign were written. This front page enabled staff coming on to shift to quickly look at the front of the folder, and see if there were any incidents that they needed to be aware of before starting their shift.

The Incident Folder enabled me to feed back more effectively to the monthly multi-disciplinary team meeting. I could develop an overall picture of what was happening with each individual and the group as a whole, without having to search in several different places. The Incident Folder held all the information regarding incidents together in one place. I still read the individual care notes and fed back the information, as these contained general information about activities, how individual people felt on that day etc. This information was important so that we could get a balanced and clearer picture of the client each month.

The incident forms were used by the psychology team to look at possible triggers, behaviour patterns etc, and helped to develop observation and recording forms for individual clients. One use of an observation and recording chart devised by the psychologist was to observe a particular client and give feedback about how he had been over a specified period of time. Staff only fedback with the client when they had a positive message to give, other feedback was recorded but not discussed with the client. After a period of time the client would remind staff when to tick his chart. He had learnt about which behaviours were challenging. Staff initially were negative about using a tick chart as these had been used before with this client and others, and they still had behaviours which were challenging. I discussed this with staff and agreed that it was not something new and innovative, but was part of a whole approach. If something works and is positive for the client then it should be used. The tick charts do fit in to how we interact and communicate with our clients. The tick chart enabled staff to regularly interact with the client positively. It helped the client feel more positive about himself and helped communication. The client did value the feedback; if he had not valued the feedback or felt that it was not genuine or consistent, then it would not have been beneficial.

Whether it is tick charts, incident forms or whatever, I found that staff needed to feel motivated to fill in forms. If staff were not sure of the relevance of the particular form this would be the form that was forgotten! Time is always a factor when filling in forms, especially after an incident when the staff are usually the most stretched supporting clients who are often distressed. It is then that staffing support for clients is most needed, but it is also when staff need to withdraw to complete the necessary forms. This dilemma is one which is still unresolved, because when the need for staffing support decreases the incident has passed, and the staff member does not always remember all the key information. Staff are encouraged to work together to record information, especially about what was happening before and during the incident. The person involved in the incident may have literally been too close to see everything and evaluate their response. It is the other staff members around who can pick up on the body language of both the member of staff and the client involved in the incident and feed this back to the staff member.

Supporting staff – Tracey Culshaw

It was important to stress to staff the importance of talking the incident over with someone as soon after the incident as possible. This was critical for staff in accessing support and ensuring good team practice. In the early days, when the team was more fragmented, it proved a vital gap of support for many staff. The staff working with the clients need to be able to work closely and confidently as a team, they need to feel safe enough with each other to be honest and to accept critical feedback positively. I found that after much team-building work and genuine effort and commitment by the staff, they were very supportive of each other, especially after an incident. When staff from other units came to work in the house, e.g. when they swapped with a member of staff who was pregnant (pregnant staff could not work in the unit), they gave very positive feedback about the team spirit and often commented on the relaxed atmosphere and humour within the team. The atmosphere of the working environment is essential as this is the atmosphere of the living environment for our clients. Our clients probably pick up on more of the non-verbal communication than we as staff do. If the atmosphere is tense and stressed, this would affect how they feel and interact. Our clients may not know why the atmosphere is tense, and may assume that it is a reflection on how we feel about them. Good teamwork led to a good working atmosphere and therefore a better environment for our clients to live in. Humour was often used and was most effective in defusing a stressful environment.

This support from staff and self-analysis means that staff are able to question whether they want to or are suited to working in this particular unit. I have always encouraged staff to discuss with myself and their colleagues the particular needs of this unit. It is not a suitable place of work for all care staff. Because it is not a suitable place for one person it does not diminish their qualities as a member of care staff. A person may be a very good carer, but not be able to communicate non-verbally effectively with a client. When we interact with clients we hope to give out positive non-verbal communication, i.e. a relaxed, approachable confident message, and this is hard to do if you feel uncomfortable or frightened of a particular person. Alternatively if you feel over confident, you may give out signals that are perceived by the client as aggressive and confrontational. It is a very difficult balance, but vital in being able to work with this particular client group. Our body language is probably the most difficult thing to see in ourselves and therefore, to control. A member of staff may interact with a client and feel they interacted very well, and be surprised by the client's reaction. We, as observers, may have noticed the confrontational body posture but getting the member of staff to see and accept this can be very difficult. One of the ways I helped staff evaluate their body language was to encourage them to discuss openly and honestly with each other what they saw. A good supportive team relationship is essential.

I've always talked openly with staff about the possibility of working in another unit if either they or I felt that they were not coping well in this particular unit. I always highlighted that this does not reflect their abilities as carers. If someone is finding it difficult it reflects in their motivation and how they perform at work. If it is just a short phase, maybe they are not feeling 100% on that day, I encourage staff to communicate this to their colleagues. They would then work in a less stressful and intense environment. Again, team skills come into play. I feel that the ability to say when you aren't at your best is a positive quality and one which I encourage the team to respect in each other. If someone was going through a series of 'bad' days or through a prolonged period of difficulty in their personal life, then I would talk with them and together we would look at what support needs they had and, ultimately, their ability to work in this unit.

The 'Meeting a Challenge' successfully provided the foundation for staff to build on. It enabled staff to begin to work as a team with shared views and consistent attitudes. The staff went on to look at different ways they could help the clients change how they felt and perceived things. The key factor was that staff were being more positive about the possible reasons for the clients' behaviour. They also acknowledged their role as an enabler and/or catalyst in changing clients' behaviour. I believe in the Rogerian outlook (Rogers 1956) that a change in behaviour will follow a change in the way a person sees themselves or how they feel about themselves. Rogers argued that given the right climate a person will 'grow'. This climate involved providing the basic core conditions of empathy, genuineness and unconditional positive regard. I believe that when interacting with our clients we must always express empathy, warmth, honesty and caring. We must 'prize' and empower our clients in our daily interactions. We must be positive, non-judgemental and approachable. It is this attitude and approach which will help our clients feel valued. I feel this is the key factor which determines the success of working with people in general, but especially in working with people with low self-esteem. When interviewing for staff this is the hardest thing to assess at interview but the most crucial attribute needed to work with this particular client group.

One particular lady I worked with used to dislike herself and continued to behave in a way that reinforced this dislike. Her dislike of herself stemmed from experiences in her past which left her feeling that she was not likeable. As staff continued to give her the message she was liked, she behaved in a more extreme manner to resolve this conflict and attempted to get staff to dislike her. It was during these difficult times that staff needed additional support. Regular staff meetings, supervision and time for staff to express how they are feeling are very important. Eventually, with support she has changed how she sees herself and this has reflected in her behaviour.

Another difficulty, which still arises, is for staff to continue to feel positive, caring and warm after an assault. It is imperative that staff have the opportunity to debrief after an incident. The manner of this debrief should be one of support for the staff, and not one in which the staff member feels their behaviour is being 'checked out'. It may be that the incident could have been avoided. For example, the staff member may have used a 'trigger' word. Of course, it is important for me to admit to the occasions where, on reflection, I said or did the wrong thing. I hope that the relationship between myself and the staff is open, warm, honest, empathic and caring too! It is during this debriefing that incident records can be made in a positive way to enable information to be analysed to develop future care plans, etc. I am aware that if the reason for this record keeping is not explained adequately, staff are left feeling that the records are to be used as a 'stick to beat them with' later.

Case study – Tracey Culshaw and Karin Purvis

To illustrate our way of working , we have written a case study.

David is a 39-year-old man with severe learning disabilities. He has lived in hospitals for people with learning disabilities and smaller residential establishments for most of his life. He attends day care for four days a week. He is a very large man, and has a long history of displaying challenging behaviours, such as hitting, kicking, biting, being verbally abusive and destroying property.

David is very talkative and has good social and expressive language. He usually speaks very clearly, and is easy to understand, although he has a tendency to shout. David has an excellent memory for past events and people he knew, and talks about these constantly. David is very sociable and enjoys meeting people. However, he tends to be 'forward' when meeting people and approaches complete strangers and familiar people in the same way. He does not respect personal space, assumes shared knowledge and finds it difficult to begin conversations appropriately. David becomes particularly anxious during periods of change, when his usual routines are different, e.g. at Christmas, during staff changes. When he is anxious he shouts, becomes verbally aggressive and finds it difficult to take on new information. These episodes often culminate in assaults on staff.

Relationships

David had difficulty in forming relationships with people. When meeting a new member of staff he immediately assumed that they did not like him and, consequently, he did not like them. David's anxieties around new staff were because he had no established relationship with them. As he would have to interact with these people on a daily basis this lack of relationship and assumption of dislike was a major problem for him and for new members of staff. David's insecurity resulted in him verbally abusing and, sometimes, physically assaulting new staff when he met them. This was particularly daunting and frightening for staff, because David was bigger than most of them! This behaviour confirmed David's reputation for being aggressive, and resulted in new staff being very wary when they met him – this was often reflected in their body language. This body language reinforced David's original belief that new staff did not like him, because he was unable to differentiate between body language of fear and dislike, and so the vicious circle continued.

Initially we tried to give David the message that the new member of staff liked him by preparing him before they started work. This was unsuccessful, because David became very anxious and it was impossible to find the right time to prepare him.

Our second strategy was successful in helping to guide the relationship building process, but did not eliminate the initial confrontation. As part of this strategy, David went out to a familiar place with a familiar person and the new member of staff. The new person was encouraged to take the lead in supporting David, for example, by helping David to order his lunch. The next time, David and the new member of staff would do the same thing again, but on their own (with a mobile phone for emergency back up). David quickly experienced the new person doing something positive with him and assumed that they liked him. The relationship between the two could then begin to develop.

However, the initial meeting was still an area of difficulty. New staff were introduced into the house at times when David was out, so that they could familiarise themselves with the other clients and the running of the Unit. This built up their confidence and gave them the opportunity to read David's care plans and acquire some knowledge about him prior to meeting him. This, in itself, was difficult to balance: staff needed to build up their confidence without building up their concerns.

The solution to the initial meeting came by chance. A new member of staff was in the office when David arrived home unexpectedly early. He immediately started to shout and ask what they were doing. The new member of staff happened to have a can of diet coke (David's favourite drink) in their hand, which they handed to him, saying 'This is for you'. David accepted the drink and the person! The 'diet coke' method of relationship building worked with a number of new staff and at times when staff from other Units provided relief cover.

Staff had to build on the initial good encounter in preparation for the time when they would have to enforce a boundary and/or say 'No'. This could be a very difficult moment, regardless of whether the relationship had been established! The fact that there was a relationship helped David move past this point and it was often possible to explain why the staff member had said 'No'. If the relationship had been new or unestablished, this would continue to be a point of conflict and David would feel that the staff permanently disliked him. It would then be much harder to overcome this, as David would have lost trust in the member of staff and his relationship with them.

Enforcing boundaries

There were a number of boundaries that had to be enforced, e.g. that David could not enter other people's bedrooms, he could not have half a bag of sugar on his breakfast cereal. Initially, David would accept boundaries, but, after a period of time or during a period of anxiety would test whether the boundary was still there, by hitting or threatening to hit staff. Unfortunately, some staff understandably were not always able to maintain the boundary, particularly if they were alone or felt threatened. This resulted in the boundary being inconsistently enforced, and so David tested it more frequently with other staff. When boundaries were consistently enforced there were no problems.

As a staff team, we had to work together on addressing this problem and stress the need for consistency, e.g. for David to be reassured he needed to know where he stood and what was expected of him and that boundaries were still in place. As a team we evaluated the boundaries which were important to maintain and why and how we could do this as a team. It took a long time to achieve this. When we got it right, the number of incidents decreased. One of the strategies used when staff were alone and felt threatened was for them to say 'I'll check' and go and get another member of staff to help.

Staff had to be able to work with the boundaries – the team was as strong as the weakest link. Staff had the opportunity to re-evaluate the boundaries and agree on whether they felt they were needed – there was no point in putting people in a vulnerable situation for something that they saw as being insignificant, e.g. David used to put his shoes on the table. Staff agreed that David's shoes should be removed and the table wiped, rather than there being a confrontation.

Calming

One of the most successful elements was the introduction of a relaxation programme. David found it very difficult to relax, and was not aware of when he was becoming anxious. A programme was devised so that when staff noticed David becoming up-tight they would suggest listening to a tape in his bedroom with him. He liked listening to tapes on a one-to-one basis. Once he was in his room we encouraged him to breathe in and out slowly. We used a relaxed tone of voice and calming words and talked about the feelings in his chest and stomach. After a relatively short time he would ask staff to come and listen to tapes with him in his room. He began to recognise the feelings of getting upset or angry and found a more effective way to relax. Before this David would hit out at people. The programme initially had two people working with him in his room, but it proved so successful it was quickly reduced to one person. If, at any time, David had to be removed from an incident we used the same programme and encouraged deep breathing and listening to relaxing music. David chose the tape he liked most, Pan Pipes, and asked to take it to work (the day centre). The same programme was then introduced to the day centre successfully.

Communication

People who knew David felt that his understanding of what was said to him was good. David was referred for speech and language therapy assessment. The assessment took the form of working with David individually and within group settings, and discussion with staff in residential, day services and the multi-disciplinary team.

Assessment indicated that David had very good understanding of situations and non-verbal cues, such as body language, facial expression and tone of voice. He had good understanding of familiar events (particularly past events and people) and was able to discuss these. At the single word level, David was able to identify familiar common objects only. In connected speech, David was able to understand sentences

123

with two or three information carrying words, provided that he was familiar with the individual words, e.g. the *spoon* is *under* the *box* the *lady* is *carrying* the *bag*.

David often remembered the first and last words only, and repeated these, to help him remember. He introduced topics that were familiar and comfortable to him when he was anxious, and often talked about these repetitively, e.g: saying, 'Simon is my key worker. He's at home today' continually for two to three hours. He would become anxious if staff changed the wording.

In addition, David showed no understanding of the word 'not', e.g. 'the dog is not drinking' was interpreted as 'the dog is drinking'. In everyday life, David had often shown confusion when negatives were used. It is likely that he became very confused, because he was picking up non-verbal cues associated with negatives, but not understanding that a negative had been used verbally. This had been masked by the fact that David used negative structures expressively.

David had very poor understanding of time concepts. He was able to label meals, but knew the days of the week according to what activities happened, e.g. market day was on Friday, art was on Thursday. If an activity changed, his ability to understand time had gone.

David's expressive language was found to be excellent. However, he often used phrases and sentences in the appropriate situation, but without understanding their meaning, e.g. 'Did you have a good car accident this morning?' when a member of staff almost had a car accident; greeting another member of staff with: 'Hello, how's your husband? Is he still dead?' David's expressive language masked his verbal comprehension difficulties. Those of us who worked with him were surprised by the level of his comprehension difficulties, and how well his difficulties had been masked.

A report outlining David's communication skills was written and distributed to the residential unit, day care and all professionals who worked with David. This included advice on presenting information to him, simplifying language and alternative ways of presenting negatives. There were some aspects which required specific communication programmes. For example, the word 'holiday' caused David enormous anxiety. David had never been on holiday, and we discovered that the word had been used, in the past, when staff had left work for ever and had wanted to avoid a confrontation with him. 'Holiday' is also a vague term and can indicate variable lengths of time.

A programme was developed which used the idea of people 'taking it in turns' to go on holiday. The person going on holiday told David that they were going the day before, and gave him information about where they were going, etc. They completed a symbol calendar with him, which indicated when they would be returning from holiday. During their absence, David crossed off the days on the calendar with other members of staff. David also received a postcard from the person while they were on holiday. David went on holiday himself for the first time, which naturally helped him to understand the concept of being on holiday. Now, David copes well with staff going on holiday, because he believes us when we say that we will be coming back.

As David has a very poor concept of time, we are still only able to prepare him for these events the day before. This has implications for staff, to ensure that David does not overhear them discussing these events.

David found negatives much easier to understand when they were presented visually. This was done in symbols, with a red cross drawn through the symbol. David quickly learnt that a red cross meant 'No'. This was reinforced verbally by using short sentences which set the subject first, followed by the negative. Sign and appropriate body language and tone of voice were important.

David today

Although David still has anxious times, there has been a marked decrease in the number of incidents. We feel sure that this is due to the work that staff have put into establishing a good relationship with David and presenting information in a way that he understands. David is more relaxed, tolerant of others and displays a wicked sense of humour! A member of staff commented recently that 'We are now seeing David the person, not David the behaviour'.

Conclusions

We are continuing to work on developing self-esteem with our clients by encouraging positive relationships and appropriate communication. Although we have had some success, several problems have been, and continue to be, encountered.

Although all staff completed the basic Somerset Total Communication training, there was a long gap between this and their being required to use these skills. This meant that knowledge had been forgotten, and that people lacked the confidence to use the skills. In retrospect, it would have been better to have run refresher courses on a regular basis. More people should have attended more advanced communication training, which covers issues around working with clients in more depth, and usually results in staff feeling more confident in using Somerset Total Communication. These people would have been able to provide encouragement and support for other staff.

Tackling the issues around people having pre-conceived ideas about clients' communication skills should have been done much earlier. It is difficult to know how this can be achieved successfully. Greater success seems to have been achieved after people were involved in a situation where an individual very clearly did not understand, and this was patently demonstrated in their behaviours. This is an issue that has still not been resolved. We are starting to develop a policy across the area whereby establishments make a formal commitment to support Somerset Total Communication and individual clients' communication programmes. This commitment is monitored closely by senior managers, and staff are made aware that this is local policy and must be adhered to.

There has been difficulty in monitoring the implementation of recommendations regarding communication across shifts, and with staff who do not believe in the validity of these recommendations. This is beginning to be addressed by the development of the local policy described above.

It is hard to maintain consistency across the staff group, family and carers, day services and the multi-disciplinary team. More objective record keeping would have been useful. We know that the changes in some individuals have been quite remarkable, but we do not have any specific records to substantiate this, other than that the number of incidents has decreased.

On reflection though, this way of working appears to have been largely successful in meeting our aims. These were to promote quality relationships, increase self-esteem and self-worth in our clients, begin to address their communication needs and provide a safe environment which staff enjoyed working in. This has been demonstrated by an increased sense of well-being in our clients, and a decrease in the number of incidents of challenging behaviour. There are still, and will continue to be, times when individuals require more intensive support. We are all becoming better at identifying these times earlier.

We feel that this success has been possible for many reasons. The development of a spacious quality environment promoted a sense of self-worth, and gave clients the space that they often needed to work through their emotions. We all have the right to display our emotions in our own home.

The presence of more appropriate record keeping has ensured that clients' behaviours are more adequately monitored and provided information that has been used in the development of care plans. This has gone hand-in-hand with strategies to provide on-going support for staff. The belief that the staff team should also support each other, has been actively promoted. Monthly multi-disciplinary team meetings have been invaluable for monitoring progress, discussing difficulties and problem solving. We all have a contribution to make to these meetings.

The staff team's great commitment to working with this group of clients during some extremely difficult times has been fundamental to this way of working.

We look forward to continuing to develop our skills in this area. We continue to learn as much from our clients as much as we teach them.

References

Calculator, S.N. (1988) 'Exploring the language of adults with mental retardation', in Calculator, S. N. and Bedrosian, J. (eds) *Communication Assessment and Intervention with Adults with Mental Retardation*. London: Taylor and Francis.

Cottam, P. J. (1986) 'Speech therapy provision and management of mentally handicapped adults', *British Journal of Mental Subnormality* **32**, 108–13.

Jones, J., Turner, J., Heard, A. (1992) 'Making communication a priority', *College of Speech and Language Therapists Bulletin*, February, 6–7.

Maslow, A. H. (1970) *Motivation and Personality*. New York: Harper and Row.

Nind, M. and Hewett, D. (1994) *Access to Communication: Developing the Basics of Communication with People with Severe Learning Difficulties Through Intensive Interaction*. London: David Fulton Publishers.

Purvis, K. (1996) 'An evaluation of the implementation of Somerset Total Communication', unpublished research project, Avalon Somerset NHS Trust.

Rogers, C. (1956) *Client-centred Therapy*. London: Constable Brown.

Somerset Total Communication Resource Base, Northgate Offices, 41–43 Northgate, Bridgwater, Somerset TA6 3EU.

Chapter 8

Andrew – a classroom for one

Maggie Roberts and Ann Vine

Maggie Roberts:

The background

Our project came about when Andrew was excluded from our school at a late stage in his school career. His levels of violence and other challenging behaviours had escalated to a point where other pupils were at such risk that this unhappy decision was felt necessary.

During the period of his exclusion Andrew's parents failed to secure an alternative placement as a consequence of his aggressive behaviours (Andrew's reputation preceded him) and they rejected residential care as the only available option. For many reasons, their desire was that he remain at home in spite of the intolerable strain. Being very protective of him, they feared him vulnerable to ill treatment as a retaliatory measure to his aggressive behaviour.

As it became clear Andrew's future was in jeopardy the head teacher (Hazel Court) stepped in, and battled to set up an educational provision as a make or break endeavour. In September 1995, after nine months at home without education, Andrew was allocated 2:1 teaching support funded by the education authority and managed through Hazel Court School in a unit attached to Chestnut Drive Children's Resource Centre. Ann Vine and myself were appointed as teaching staff and contracted to work with Andrew for 15 months.

Andrew is five feet seven inches and of a fairly stocky build, possessing considerable physical strength. Naturally, this contributed both to his challenging ability and his reputation for it. Andrew has autism and functions at a level of profound learning difficulties, though he is mobile, albeit with a slightly awkward gait.

Ann Vine – teaching assistant

When I first met Andrew at his school he was 15 years old and in a class of six pupils. Although certainly the biggest he was not always the most troublesome. However, Andrew's final year at school before exclusion had been difficult for him and for the staff. I, too, was saddened by his exclusion and so, when it was decided to appoint a teacher and teaching assistant to work with Andrew, I applied.

Maggie (with whom I had worked briefly in the past) was appointed teacher

127

with myself as the teaching assistant. Maggie was trained as a mainstream primary school teacher and, although she had done some supply work in a severe learning difficulties (SLD) school, she was not experienced in autism or challenging behaviour.

My previous career was totally unconnected with special needs education, but since being appointed to Hazel Court School I had already gained 'one to one' experience with another child, albeit in totally different, non-violent, circumstances.

Despite some apprehension, I felt that we were suitable to take on this task. We both thought that a fresh approach with no preconceptions could succeed, together with some appropriate training. The fact that several experts in various specialised fields, working with Andrew on an *ad hoc* basis, had made no appreciable progress made us optimistic that a full-time commitment could be more successful, particularly as this approach had not been tried before. Andrew was nine months into his exclusion when the project commenced. Premises had not yet been arranged and we were required to work initially from his home.

We were stunned at the degree of regression in Andrew's behaviour over these nine months. He would shout, roar and stamp continually, combining this with spitting, hissing and wringing his hands. The hair at the back of his head had been worn down by the rubbing action of being continually in bed. He was totally caught up in ritualistic behaviour and ignored us completely. Maggie was certainly not prepared for this and has since admitted that at this first meeting she too was shocked.

Our initial approach was to really get to know Andrew and to re-gain his trust. Our relationship with his parents was good. Their bitterness towards the school did not extend to us and they were very hospitable and really relieved that Andrew's education was being resumed. They were further heartened by the fact that we were not frightened of him and demonstrated a genuine concern for his welfare. Their expectations for him were simple. They wanted him to be happy, go swimming, to learn a few self help skills and, above all, to remain with them as part of the family.

Working from Andrew's home proved impossible despite his parents' full co-operation. Being at home meant that he was able to stay in his room for as long as he wished with no element of pressure to extend his abilities. He appeared unable to differentiate between the relaxed atmosphere of home and the challenging environment of a school situation.

Andrew had developed a determined preference for riding in a wheelchair, even though he was perfectly able to walk naturally. He enjoyed being taken for walks but would resist any attempt to coax him from the wheelchair by lashing out over his shoulder.

At this time we were severely restricted by the delay in authorising the use of our private cars which meant that we could only make daily excursions on foot. We would constantly cover the same route resulting in little fresh stimulation for Andrew.

Andrew's parents were keen to see a greater volume of schoolwork, despite

Maggie's judgement that this would be unsuitable for the home environment. An attempt at playing a game on the dining room table resulted in such a violent outburst that they accepted that no real progress would be made until proper premises had been arranged.

Premises became an absolute priority. Andrew needed a new start. We were intruding on his territory in his home and this put the whole project in jeopardy. Finally, a chance encounter with a staff member of a nearby Children's Resource Centre resulted in two rooms with kitchen and bathroom facilities being made available. We named our new premises 'Rainbow House'. A separate entrance ensured that Andrew, who also attends the Resource Centre, would not connect his school situation with his respite care.

Maggie Roberts:

Andrew's psychological condition at the beginning of the project

At the start of the project Andrew's condition could be described as follows:

- inward looking and deeply involved in self-stimulatory activities;
- little self control in terms of behaviour (violent rages at home), impatient and unable to wait for anything, particularly food;
- intolerant of the activity of people around him;
- closed down in terms of little to no reaction to his external environment;
- passive in terms of self-help skills – would attempt very little for himself;
- physically lazy, preferred to sit in a wheelchair (the wheelchair had become his focus of interest);
- short concentration span;
- limited eye contact;
- lots of angry communications more often than not a cloudy countenance;
- withdrawn socially.

At home

According to Andrew's father, Andrew resisted his family entering into 'his personal space'. He was solitary, spending much time in his own bedroom. In the evenings, his pattern was to go to bed early, never joining the family in the sitting room (with the exception of rocking in the doorway and throwing objects into the room). He reacted adversely to strangers coming into the home, particularly workmen who came to extend the bathroom over a lengthy period. During the building work Andrew's problematic behaviour escalated.

The Chestnut Drive situation (the resource centre for respite care)

Only two workers would happily work with Andrew, both of whom were men. In the worst periods, the two staff had to work back-to-back shifts when Andrew was in for respite care. At Chestnut Drive, Andrew's preference was either his bedroom or the large open space of the playroom. He declined to stay in the unit with the rest of the children and staff, and resisted entering into the activities on offer.

The structure of the terms (September 95–December 97)

Mum was predominantly the most important character in Andrew's life. We used this relationship to gain access to a friendship with Andrew. We initially embarked on a visiting period. Visiting twice weekly, our time usually spent out walking, we established in Andrew's eyes a friendship between ourselves and his mother – no pressure was put on him. We remained quite background figures, giving him ample time simply to adjust to our physical presence. This strategy provided an opportunity for assessment (mum also supplied us with information) and had the added advantage of tying us in with his favourite activity. After two weeks of visiting we ventured out minus mum – this presented no problems.

Chestnut Drive: Second half of the September term 1995 to 19th December 1997

Finally we were installed at Chestnut Drive. We were linked to our school and drew support from there. Andrew embraced his new environment and explored day one.

Initially, we presented very little in terms of stimulus in the rooms, affording time for Andrew to adjust to the physical environment itself. Over time the rooms grew correspondingly to Andrew's development (a very visual classroom was envisaged). The daily timetable evolved also in accordance with Andrew's needs and remained flexible. Due attention was paid to Andrew's preferences, i.e. he enjoyed swimming so we swam twice a week. As well as the hydrotherapy pool at Chestnut Drive we went to a public swimming pool – another milestone in achievement. He exhibited preferences for walking in certain places, so our planning incorporated those preferences. In these early stages little pressure was placed on Andrew in terms of educational activities. Activities were conducted at his pace and set at his tempo. Our main concern was relationship building and setting up conditions for optimal learning. A slowly, slowly approach was the cornerstone. We continuously recorded Andrew's behaviour as this was a priority. No substantial intervention was planned until a greater understanding of Andrew as an individual was secured.

Term 2

We experienced an initial set-back after the holiday period and due adjustment was made. This was not experienced again after a holiday break, representing a greater consolidation of gains. However, the rapport now seemed established and with Andrew settled, the time was optimal to move on and extend Andrew's abilities. Our main focus thereafter was on three issues: more actively reducing the negative behaviour, teaching Andrew new strategies for communicating, and providing more opportunities for socialisation.

Secondary issues included encouraging Andrew to be more active in a plethora of simple skills such as: Andrew to hang up his coat, to help put shopping in the basket. When successful, these activities had the additional advantage of allowing Andrew less time for disruptive behaviour. Our intentions also included building up a repertoire of interactive games and dealing with negative self-stimulatory practice.

Term 3

There was a continuation and extension of the work started in term 2. Also, a new dimension was incorporated in our work – the beginning of integration into adult services. This whole period was fraught with tension and difficulties, the service needing much adaptation to fit Andrew's needs. We began a once-weekly visit as part of an integration programme. We revisited with success some educational activities that Andrew would not tolerate during term 1.

Term 4

There was further development of the work from previous terms and the appointment of new staff to work with Andrew, initially alongside existing staff and then, from January 1997, to take over management of Andrew completely. Easing the change-over of staffing was the main focus of this term.

Our approach

Aims

The aims of our project were:

- to help Andrew to be easier to be with;
- to enhance Andrew's communicative abilities through extended use of gesture;
- to enable him to exact more control over his environment and to diminish

the anxiety caused by lack of understanding of the course of events during the school day;

- to encourage Andrew to be an active participant in his learning;
- to increase Andrew's tolerance levels, particularly his ability to wait;
- to encourage Andrew to self-regulate – to encourage change through his own volition, and not through coercion, by using praise, warmth, affection, physical contact, soothing tones of voice to calm legitimate distress, responding to his moods, and firm use of 'No';
- to introduce Andrew to different social settings without disruption and to extend his life experience;
- to provide alternatives to anti-social self-stimulatory activities;
- to prepare Andrew for adult services;
- to synthesise, use and document procedures, practices and techniques for the above;
- to pass on and advocate to future staff good and effective procedures, practices and techniques.

Establishing a rapport

Relationship building was considered to be the most important aspect on which the whole approach was underpinned. Initially the welfare of staff was sacrificed to achieve this. Staff sustained innumerable injuries, i.e. bruising to arms, for two reasons: to work intensively with Andrew and to convey to Andrew an unconditional acceptance of him as an individual.

By term 2 as the relationship seemed sufficiently formed, conditions in terms of acceptable behaviour were gradually introduced, and a more balanced relationship evolved. In the negotiation of this it was crucial to have an understanding of autism and the effects of profound learning difficulties on the individual.

Child-centred

A highly individualised timetable developed. Working at Andrew's pace and tempo was recognised as essential, as was offering an optimal environment; slowly introducing Andrew to an increasingly visual environment with display work and other materials of stimulus. The environment was initially spartan to avoid detracting from the key aspect of familiarising Andrew with the physical layout and atmosphere of the building. Personalising the setting was a feature, i.e. wall space was dedicated to photographs of Andrew, which also provided a visual commentary of the activity of the year.

Cognitively speaking, activities were set that were achievable and meaningful, emphasis was placed on increasing Andrew's understanding of the world and himself as an operator in it, and particularly on creating opportunities for Andrew to self-regulate his behaviour.

Short-term strategies to behaviour management were introduced, with the long-term approach involving building communicative alternatives. We always operated on the basis that his challenging behaviour was an immature method of communicating his feelings.

The 'Intensive Interaction' approach had its role. Particularly successful were short interactive games such as 'cheek popping' – the notion of tasklessness' was appropriate at times. Imitating Andrew's actions and sounds met with little success and often with hostility, particularly reproducing one sound that was very personal to him.

The management of incidents

Details of incident management procedures

The underlying principle to all behaviour management was 'How can I help this person to retain or regain self control?' The secondary aim was to use all these situations to further Andrew's understanding of himself and other people. As far as possible, behaviour concerns were not limiting us in what we wished Andrew to experience, within the boundaries of his disability and the need for safety. We worked with a positive expectation of positive behaviour by Andrew.

The response to an incident was often highly intuitive, but based on a framework of practices and procedures developed from an understanding and knowledge of Andrew as an individual and the nature of his emotions and disabilities.

Key features

We focused on prevention and redirection and increasingly developed our own clear guidelines for challenging situations, particularly when out:

- initial assessment of situation (we formed a highly-developed sensitivity to the environment as a result of working with Andrew);
- calming techniques – reassurance, removal of stress – if anxiety induced spoken or unspoken communication between staff;
- effective signalling to other parties.

Action entailed:

- use of language, i.e. key words, sameness of language, a phrase continually repeated;
- non-verbal communication – at times this was more useful as Andrew has quite a speedy comprehension of explicit or exaggerated non-verbal communication;

133

- redirection, if possible use of any available practical structures, i.e. a seat;
- use of space;
- use of time;
- removal or limitation of exposure to trigger;
- ensuring the environment is as safe as possible, i.e. avoidance of any area with glass – Andrew has a tendency to aim for glass;
- a degree of physical holding (for which we were trained) if necessary to prevent damage to self, staff or others (as advocated by the Loddon School adapted from SCIP/OMRDD/NY/USA)
- making sure the incident ends on a positive note for Andrew;
- extracting the learning in the aftermath and presenting it to Andrew in an accessible manner.

Examples of incidents

Three incidents should be considered together, falling during 11–29 March 1996. This period was a prolonged build-up to a seizure, although we were unaware of this initially. We had experienced pre-seizure build-up on two previous occasions, but not of this magnitude or duration. As we progressed through this phase we were searching for explanations for the deterioration in his mood state, theorising that perhaps in this closing stage of term, over-tiredness was the central element. It was interesting how the period developed, one part of the day being problematical, seemingly following a pattern, and then equilibrium being restored.

Incident no. 1: Monday 11 March
Andrew had spent the weekend at Chestnut Drive as part of his respite package. The trigger to his difficult behaviour had occurred on his way to the Rainbow rooms. The unit we occupied was an integral part of the Chestnut complex, but we established it as a separate entity in Andrew's eyes through the use of the outside entrance. The passing of my car had instilled in Andrew a desire to get in it, and when this was denied, it provoked an angry outburst towards the Chestnut staff.

Later, in the Rainbow rooms, ill humour was apparent and remained unabated by breakfast, which further served to fuel the hostile mood – the breakfast plate was pushed away for 'finished' untouched (a late first breakfast can be assumed). Great agitation ensued with furniture pushed and knocked over amid angry and challenging vocalisations, the furore including hitting and pinching, standard behaviour in these situations.

Andrew went to get his coat, the car still being uppermost in his mind. Ann and I didn't feel this demand could be met, his mood was so volatile it would have been hazardous in the car. An attempted shout-down met with no success. We ushered Andrew out into a safer environment – the outside courtyard – then backed off and monitored the situation. Time passed, self-control was seemingly restored. Andrew held out his hand to request our daily outing. We responded, but as a safeguard, initially walked around the neighbouring vicinity. Deeming the situation resolved – Andrew by this point was trying to manoeuvre us towards nearby cars, irrespective of any resemblance to our own vehicle – we ventured to our own car. Andrew sat peacefully throughout the journey after having tolerated staff incompetence in taking several attempts to fasten up his seat belt.

Incident no. 2: Thursday 14 March

Breakfast time, or more precisely the first part of the day, was increasingly becoming an agitated time, a pattern being established (previously this had been a most relaxed period). Immediately following breakfast Andrew expressed a desire to go out by fetching his coat and we helped him put it on. A few minutes delay was occasioned by the need for Ann and I to put our coats on. This lack of immediate gratification triggered a tremendous outburst: hitting, banging, the front door window was smashed during the rumpus, and flapping of hands quite clearly indicated a displeased Andrew. In response we carefully relieved him of his jacket to signal the unlikelihood of us venturing out should the outburst continue, alongside a verbal commentary of similar ilk, delivered in a calm tone. Further steps were required to lower the emotional tone. Andrew was again ushered outside and left to cool off. When he appeared calmer, I held out a hand to him. Initially the proffered hand was refused, but after a short re-think the invitation was accepted. The remainder of the day passed pleasurably without a re-occurrence of trouble.

Incident no. 3: Wednesday 20 March

The next outburst was centred around coffee time, although an ill-humoured mood was apparent from the beginning of the day, as was a distinct lack of any initiation of positive interaction.

During coffee Andrew had requested more cake. As the cake was finished, biscuits were offered as an alternative. Andrew misread staff intentions and took a biscuit from the plate instead of the plate itself, which was his. When asked to try again he threw the biscuit on the floor. A few minutes later biscuits were re-offered with the same request to take the plate. This instigated an outburst followed by a charge into the hall to obtain his coat and an attempted departure via the front door. At this point we requested that he should sit on the waiting chair, hoping to serve the dual purpose of containing his rage, but also signalling the future possibility of an outing when calm was restored. However, his high state of arousal was not to be diffused at this point and an angry scene developed, Andrew head butting and lashing out at staff and property. Procedures used on similar occasions were put into practice, i.e. Andrew went outside.

During the 20–29 March Andrew's behaviour followed much the same pattern: banging and shouting the hallmark of waiting for breakfast; increasing intolerance being displayed in situations that previously had been managed well; extreme mood swings becoming the norm, the transition between one and the other effected within seconds. Andrew's ability to self-regulate declined rapidly. The offering of cake at coffee time, until recently a favourite time of the day developed into a new trigger as a consequence of incident no. 3. The fetching of his coat to indicate the desire to go out became in his eyes the panacea for all ills. The level of Andrew's social interaction dropped dramatically. Activities were suspended unless they were low risk, anything representing a challenge to Andrew was avoided. On 30 March Andrew had two seizures followed a few days later in the half term holiday by several more.

Evaluation

The period was very thought provoking as well as extremely exhausting, particularly towards the end when Ann and myself felt wholly depleted of stamina. Seizures can represent a time of extreme difficulty for staff and the individual alike. Judging from this last experience it would appear that in the initial stages staff could be very effective in helping Andrew to manage his behaviour, but as the seizure became imminent on a prolonged build-up, Andrew's ability to self-regulate declined as the internal pressure became too intense for him to cope with.

Because of the levels of agitation an indoor environment was more hazardous for Andrew's safety and that of staff. Ushering Andrew outside eliminated damage to himself, property and staff. The fresh air too acting literally and metaphorically as a cooling down' agent meant that staff were able to move to a safe distance, ceasing to be a stimulus and to monitor the situation. Andrew was left without interference to regain his equilibrium. When faced with inclement weather our practice was to use the upstairs bedroom, as lying on the bed had a calming effect on Andrew's behaviour.

Andrew modified his behaviour in the light of experience, making attempts to rectify situations and restore conviviality. Incidents 1 and 2 aimed at conveying to Andrew that as soon as he was calm following an outburst staff would respond to his requests. The waiting chair was introduced in response to incident no. 2 and has proved to be effective over a long period.

On reflection from incidents earlier in the year, we had become more efficient at dealing with crises. We had sought to soothe in a conventional manner, i.e. soothing talk and touch (there is a place for this at anxiety times but not in high arousal). At higher levels touching had acted as a stimulus, prolonging the state of agitation.

Range of possible incidents

Incidents could manifest themselves in either the external or internal environment irrespective of situation or setting. The most insignificant or even pleasurable event in normal terms (particularly an unpredictable one) could bring about overload, for example a chance bumping into Andrew's parents in an unexpected place. Other triggers included: anxiety situations; not understanding why a visitor hasn't already departed; intolerance, e.g. having to wait; certain noises – in particular a baby's cry; self-stimulatory activity (rocking), could induce a high state of arousal; or even a simple demand made upon him in the form of a request, e.g. being asked to hang his coat up. Minor incidents could have the capacity to develop into major ones depending on the general mood state. Vulnerable times, especially the pre-seizure build-up, were hazardous as Andrew's tolerance level was lowered generally. Incidents fluctuated between minor skirmish type scenarios in a setting such as in Tesco supermarket – hitting, pinching and shouting (triggered by having to wait – he actually does like Tesco!). A similar situation on Eastbourne sea front triggered by the cry of a seagull, to a prolonged full-scale rampage at Chestnut Drive, confrontational vocalisations accompanied by the shaking of arms and head, lashing out at staff, self-injurious behaviour, bashing windows and slamming doors, overturning tables, and the ultimate response of throwing himself on the floor and biting.

Recording

Record keeping was of paramount importance as all major management strategies were devised as a result of our data. The daily writing and discussions also helped to clarify our thinking and entrenched Andrew's behaviours deeply into our thoughts aiding spontaneity of action in difficult situations.

We recorded continuously to develop an understanding of Andrew's behaviour. This involved identifying the background to his behaviour, what Andrew gained by his behaviour, e.g. terminating an aversive situation, and staff response; the quality of the behaviour, i.e. hit, pinch or gouge, and the intensity of the action. We were constantly striving to refine and develop the recording to obtain a more accurate picture. The difficulty was sometimes recording a true reflection of the day in a succinct manner. Accounting for variables presented problems. Also, the question of how to measure a 'good' day was a problem – some days subjectively speaking might have felt like a good day, but on a score level the figures were not compliant. Furthermore, did a 'good' day occur because Andrew was managing better or because Ann and I were? We included visual accounts, e.g. graphs which gave us a quick overview and a calendar, colour-coded to establish patterns. Totals could be misleading in that there might only have been three incidents of hitting on one day, but the incidents consisted of barrages of blows that raised overall scores.

The highest recorded score was 40 incidents of hits, pinches, and gouges, the lowest six. The scores fell dramatically during the first term or thereabouts, suggesting we were having positive impact on Andrew's behaviour patterns. This steadied with a slight decline there after. The severity of the blows we received substantially reduced, indicating further inroads into self-control – both quantity and quality of blows were affected.

We used the STAR model as represented by Zarkowska and Clements (1994) as an aid to behaviour analysis.

Developing communication

Andrew's communicative style

Andrew mainly uses physical prompting of people around him, for example, pushing someone's hand towards the desired object, natural gesture and eye gaze as well as negative communications such as hitting, pinching, scratching. His communication system seems limited to the 'here and now' and is context bound.

Expressive communication

In non – verbal communication, Andrew:

- always makes eye contact when he wants to 'talk' to us;
- expresses his identity in the world, 'I'm here', by shouting and shaking his head;
- vocalises at various levels of pitch and tone depending on the message and mood state;
- laughs and giggles – complemented by happy facial expression accompanied sometimes by twirling, hand flapping, wringing of hands – when in a happy state;
- shows lots of physical contact when happy, e.g. he puts his arms around members of staff's neck, kisses – the sound of a kiss in return satisfies – has a loving expression towards members of staff;
- shows increased volume of vocalisation, a different tone, challenging facial expression (head generally tilted to the side) in the angry state;
- pushes staff away when he doesn't want contact – he will also turn his back on staff.

Communication priorities developed for Andrew

At the beginning of the project Andrew relied heavily on other people reading his moods, desires and preferences. His primary communicative resource was hitting.

Our agenda for working on communication comprised:

- making ourselves as interesting as possible to activate the inner drive to communicate to 'show him there is a pay-off for communicating' using the topics Andrew was most motivated about and functionally relevant to him (communicative temptations);
- making our communication more effective; developing the use of non verbal communication;
- building up Andrew's communication system – using natural gesture and objects of reference – to provide alternatives to hitting;
- imputing intentionality to Andrew's actions;
- working hard to make language more comprehensible to him by modifying and unifying our own (much of his hitting out stemmed from poor

comprehension of language leading to uncertainty and anxiety). Getting consistency in this aspect of our work was so much easier with a team of two. Following Watson *et al.* (1989) we planned to do this partly by cutting down on verbal language or cutting it out altogether. Using more physical prompting and general cues sometimes seems to have a calming effect on such students by conveying the teachers expectations in a more understandable way (Watson *et al.* 1989).

Before February 1997 positive communication remained unrecorded (our primary focus was reducing negative behaviour). Data reflected that Andrew's communicative repertoire consisted mainly of negative communications. However, by February 1997 a noticeable shift was evident and the potential to record positive communications was logged.

Use of language by staff during incidents

'For the less able pupil with Autism, the mere use of language as a source of instruction can be a source of difficulty' (Jordan and Powell 1995: 74). We acknowledged that skilful use of language is critical to enable a child with autism to comprehend the speakers intent.

We recognised that in general our use of language needed to be explicit, literal, based on the here and now, including emphasis on key words, sparse use of language and exaggerated tone and intonation (running commentary elicited hitting, as Andrew was unable to process the information with sufficient speed). This was even more imperative during incidents when Andrew's arousal was going up. Careful judgements were necessary, about the appropriate verbal tactic for each situation based on our knowledge and understanding of Andrew.

For example, during an Asda shopping incident in December 1997, in the final stages of our work with Andrew, he was accompanied by his new staff. As we entered the store Andrew switched into one of his favourite spitting behaviours. We went into a familiar coping routine of attempting to soothe and alleviate anxiety. This seemed to be going well and Andrew appeared outwardly relaxed, happy to stop and look, and assist with putting goods into the basket.

On the homeward stretch of the Asda layout a young child let out a piercing cry. In response Andrew hit his own head, then a member of staff. We held onto Andrew either side, not in a strong grip but in our customary supportive way, progressing in this manner towards the checkout. One member of staff gave out intermittent reassurances (voice quality soft and gentle, repetitive phrases used) directly into his ear, which could have been dangerous due to the risk of being head-butted. This paid off, though, as it was visibly evident that Andrew was listening. Through this method we had effectively communicated reassurance to Andrew.

Andrew's development and progression was evident in this exchange. In the early days the pressure of this trigger necessitated a quick exit (often under a barrage of blows), but in this instance there was one hit only and Andrew had calmed (recovery time is now much quicker) before we reached the checkout. At the checkout he smiled at two women and helped unload three items of shopping on to the conveyor belt.

The incident highlighted several factors. Andrew's self-control was much greater, he was coping with the environment in a more positive manner, his level of trust in staff had increased, and he was more able to respond to their directives. Evaluating staff response to crisis, we felt that we had become more skilful in responding to meet Andrew's need, more successful as communicators, and more experienced in adopting the correct strategies.

After leaving the shop we praised Andrew most enthusiastically – we were delighted. The incident was then revisited in terms of commentary as an aid to Andrew developing a greater understanding of his ability to cope with his feelings.

The usefulness of teaching some specifics of communication

It was the pupil's Christmas lunch at Hazel Court on 15 December 1995. It was early in the project still, but we wanted Andrew to attend this event, so we decided to 'go for it'. In the midst of a noisy dining room scenario Andrew had eaten the first course of his Christmas lunch. The call now was for second helpings. Ann and I made a presumption based on his enormous appetite that Andrew would like seconds. He endeavoured to eat more and then became upset. We attempted to calm him, not with great effectiveness initially, finally removing his plate (this was early days in the development of staff management of Andrew and the identification of the difficulty). The outcome of that scenario was an action plan to teach Andrew to gesture for 'more' and 'finished' in a mealtime context.

Gesturing for 'more' and 'finished'
We decided to teach the actions of lifting and handing over the plate for 'more', pushing away the plate for 'finished' – to be accomplished in three stages:

- hand over hand, lifting up the plate plus verbal prompt;
- verbal invitation own action plus prompt;
- own action no prompt possible invitation.

Andrew found the action for 'more' easier to produce than the action for 'finished', the acquisition of the latter taking longer to achieve. His motivation too, to ask for 'more' was substantially greater! Each request for 'more' was accepted for many months. Andrew at times having maximums of six pieces of toast or three pieces of cake, our primary concern being to endorse the value of communication (limitations were imposed eventually). The sense of achievement was clearly visible in his manner and facial expression, giggles and laughter would often proceed the request for 'more'.

Gesturing for 'more' and 'finished' became a landmark accomplishment for Andrew. The real benefits derived not solely in the context of this situation but in the confidence this inspired in Andrew in his skills as a communicator and his delight in being successful. The consolidation of skills was reached in three months although by 7 February Andrew gestured for 'more' without an invitation or prompt for the first time.

Andrew spontaneously generalised this skill to his home environment and his time of respite care at Chestnut Drive. The transference of skills into other settings was extremely valuable, but perhaps more importantly the acquisition of new skills inspired confidence in others working alongside Andrew who were now confronted with concrete evidence of change. Andrew still had the potential to learn – this also had major positive implications in terms of his behaviour. The concept of 'more' and 'finished' was extended to all work situations.

Resume on the improvements in Andrew's communication

Gradually, hitting other people ceased to be a communicative first resource. In day-to-day communicative exchange and when situations were challenging for him, Andrew chose to communicate more positively. This was a major departure from his previous communication norm (we must also bear in mind the communicative effectiveness of hitting, in that it produces a desired response in others very rapidly).

This underlined two aspects in Andrew's communicative development. Firstly, that he felt more in control of situations (less anxiety through greater comprehension), and secondly that he had more communicative resources at his disposal. He had acquired taught skills (a major accomplishment for someone with profound learning difficulties and whose motivation to learn was previously low) and that he was endeavouring to test out more strategies of his own making. A further achievement was that Andrew was able to generalise these new skills into different situations.

Andrew developed a greater understanding of the pleasurable aspect of communicative exchange (he wanted to communicate with many of the people he met and expected it to be pleasant) and the value of positive communication, i.e. his needs were met and he received praise from others. He felt empowered as a communicator and his self-esteem rose.

Highs and lows

Feelings and morale – Ann Vine, teaching assistant

It is probably true to say that a project of this nature, which is so intense and insular, would be impossible if the two staff did not get on well. We were together all day, every day. There were no coffee or lunch breaks away from each other. We worked as a close-knit team and could almost sense what the other was thinking. We relied on each other for support and, on occasion, protection. At least one of us had to be 100 per cent fit at all times. We do balance each other; Maggie the eternal optimist and myself more down to earth. We share the same aims and ideals and the same outlook on life.

From the outset we were confident of success and this is still the case. There have been some low times, such as the frustration created by the belief that we would never be provided with accommodation. Only a mutual sense of humour enabled us to appreciate the sheer absurdity of the situation. Teasing from old colleagues and jokes about the staffroom (our refuge in the early days) being our office served to strengthen the bond between us.

The most distressing aspect of the project was the continual injuries resulting in a number of scars and bruises. The painful pinches to my arms caused me the most distress whereas, in Maggie's case, it was the scarring to her hands. Our lowest point occurred during the third week at Rainbow House. Andrew had settled in well, without anxiety, and was apparently enjoying himself. Our arms at this stage were already black with bruises and the thought of further injury was too much to bear. One particular entry in my diary for that week read: 'Went to bathroom. Would have stopped for a weep but no time'. We were under real pressure. I couldn't leave Maggie alone with Andrew for too long. Another entry read, 'I cannot stand this pain for a whole year' and words like 'weak', 'depressed' and 'doubts' appeared regularly that week. 'Do I even like Andrew?' was my most alarming entry. Of course, I carried on because I did like him, very much in fact – it had just been a bad day.

That same week included the only incident of friction between Maggie and myself. We nearly fell out over the backing of a display board. Maggie wanted perfection whereas I wanted speed. Tension rose and I ripped the paper off the board. Nothing was said. We got over it and have got on really well ever since.

There has always been an air of tension when we are out. Our early trips to cafes were brief affairs. We swallowed scalding coffee in our haste to be ready when Andrew decided he wished to leave, as we couldn't risk a scene. Even in the later stages we had to be prepared for any eventuality and be constantly aware of our responsibilities.

As far as the future is concerned, Maggie and I feel that we have developed a high level of expertise in the extremes of challenging behaviour. The various courses we attended were excellent and genuinely useful helping us in our day-to-day efforts. This work is extremely rewarding and exciting and we both see our future as being in this part of the field.

Maggie Roberts:

Unsuccessful targeting

We found that two main areas of minimal success in targeting warranted review, one in the area of communication, the other in that of tolerance building.

Communication

Our endeavours to introduce Andrew to a more complex system of communication through the medium of pictures in addition to the one he himself had learnt, that of gesturing for his needs and his preferences to be made known, met with little success. A factor was probably our expectation that Andrew needed to be able to do it, not matching with the present reality of his abilities – Andrew's long-term reaction to pictures and picture books had been to alternate between mouthing them and wringing them with his hands.

Also, the timescale available to introduce and develop this system as a significant feature of his communication repertoire proved to be inadequate. Other considerations took precedence or simply overwhelmed us. We had hoped to introduce Andrew to the use of pictures as a means of communication by the second half of the first term. However, the management of negative behaviours was all consuming during that period (managing Andrew on a daily basis in addition to continuously recording his behaviour, analysing our findings, and developing strategies to enable him to self-regulate and us to assist in that process). The preferred starting point – the introduction of new gesturing skills and the extension of existing ones – affording time to instigate and consolidate these aims, constituted two terms' work.

The pressing need for a communication system which would positively enhance the quality of Andrew's life and that of his carers, who suffer the consequences of the more negative aspects of Andrew's communicative attempts, perhaps overrode a sounder judgement of the real possibilities of achievement. This aspiration was also fuelled by an optimistic outlook generated by growing accomplishments in other areas.

Lack of success was not absolute; Andrew has learned to look at pictures in picture books with some pleasure, his looking facilitated by our learning to present the pictures at eye level. The mouthing and wringing of such materials has substantially diminished. Matching picture to object has not as yet been worked upon except in one area. Under the inspiration of the TEACCH course (see Mesibov *et al.* 1988) which we attended in the middle the spring term, we presented Andrew, while he was seated on the 'waiting chair' (thereby ensuring the reference to be meaningful and immediate to him) with a picture of my car, an object of most significance to him. He was asked to look and help place it back in the designated pocket. Andrew did look when requested to do so, did help to replace the picture (at great speed when disinterested), however, in spite of this, efforts in this area were discontinued. The possibilities of progression and development in the whole field of communication through pictures within the time limitations were too low to warrant further input. As for outings, Andrew complies easily with a verbal invitation, and he himself has effected an efficient means to request an outing – he simply gets his coat.

Tolerance building

This concerns the ability to walk by my car to Chestnut Drive (as stated previously we are a unit within the Chestnut Drive complex – we use external entrances and exits only) without hitting out at staff. This is a twice-weekly enterprise; one visit to the Snoezelen room the other to the hydrotherapy pool; both activities Andrew thoroughly enjoys.

However well-presented in terms of communication (i.e. verbal explanations, encouraging sounds and gestures, object references) the passing of my car or any other vehicle in a similar spot remains a hazardous affair.

One can conclude that Andrew's negative reaction was not sourced by anxiety (i.e. he didn't understand what was happening, or, that he disliked the proposed activities) but that his overriding interest was in the car. Andrew was fixed solely on the immediacy of the desired object, the purpose of our walk temporarily lost to his thinking. Running the gauntlet twice weekly was a highly undesirable activity for us. Several tactics had their origin in response to this dilemma. One was to drive straight to the Chestnut Drive main entrance at the conclusion of our daily outing. The outcome of this strategy on its initial trial was one hit rather than a smattering of blows (the norm) – Andrew reacting to the unpredictability the departure from the usual routine occasioned. Another tactic on the operations board, still untried at the time of writing, is to take an alternative route, circling around the back of the complex. Finally, the tactic was to concede – get into the car, drive the ten yards, and hope Andrew would disembark despite the brevity of the journey.

Improvements in relating to other people

By February 1997 a significant shift in terms of the frequency of positive communications was filtering through as a result of the therapeutic nature of the whole approach and the building up of communicative alternatives. The relationship with Ann and myself seemed to be generalising to the manner in which Andrew related to other people. The first seeds were visible in the Spring of 1997. Our kitchen was sometimes a through way for Chestnut staff and visitors to reach the meetings room, which was located upstairs in our unit. Staff were always apologetic at this disruption, fearing ill consequences for us. However, this situation ultimately worked to our advantage. Andrew became alert to this human traffic. Once, his attention captured, he tracked one person's whole route through. He began to vocalise and reach out and touch people as they passed.

By March, rough and tumble play, one of Andrew's favourite pastimes was possible without Andrew slipping into high arousal and becoming aggressive (carefully monitored of course – there is a point for the knowing eye at which to scale down). This we took as evidence of greater self-control and a more relaxed state of being.

On walks, the first outward sign of a developing interaction with his world was an interest in objects in the environment. This became extended to include people.

Andrew would reach out and touch other people on walks as a result of a developing expectancy of positive encounters. On 18 June a man on the Downs stopped to say hello. He approached in a very warm, positive and confident manner. Andrew equalled that approach, responded equally positively, smiling and turning back to look as the man went on his way (this type of action had only so far been a feature of his interest in cars). Other examples included Andrew smiling at two elderly ladies who passed us on our walk on 8 July in Rye and, when we stopped for coffee on 17 July, initiating contact with the waiter, a complete stranger, by touching his arm and then asking for a head rub.

The social response in coffee shops was significant. Andrew's coffee shop performance initially was food-orientated only – impatience for food was standard. Once the food was finished, departure had to be imminent. We became accustomed to burnt throats from rapid coffee drinking, as well as sustaining hits and pinches. However, as time progressed Andrew became enlivened by the social stimulus afforded by the coffee shop scenario and would often re-position himself to get a more panoramic view of the setting

Term 3 saw the introduction of Sandy Ramdas (speech therapist) and Roger Noble (clinical psychologist) who undertook weekly sessions with Andrew. Andrew accepted this new dimension to the routine at Chestnut Drive. He accepted other people working with him and became comfortable with them, asking for head rubs.

Improvements in relating at home were noted, Andrew spending more time downstairs with the family. A new development altogether occurred. Andrew would come downstairs to investigate when someone came to the door. His mother noted that for the first time Andrew had a disappointed look on his face when his brothers went out. His father commented that Andrew enjoyed rough and tumble again. His 'personal space' was no longer fiercely protected. Toleration of other people was evident: workmen came to the house again and this was not problematic; and visits to the dentist and the hairdressers were tolerable. Andrew seemed to be fully embracing a new lifestyle. He was happy to get out of bed in the morning (previously he had poor motivation to get out of bed) and he couldn't wait for the taxi to arrive.

At Chestnut Drive in the respite care situation, the change was noticeable. Andrew spent more time in the unit with everyone else and, new to this situation, became interested in people who came into the unit – reaching out to touch and vocalising (Andrew was previously oblivious to visitors). Staff were becoming more relaxed around him and lots of positive comments came forward. One member of staff, Frank, described jovially the old pattern of staff reaction towards Andrew. If he approached Andrew, the inner reaction was a desire to jump back in anticipation of an expected hit. Andrew developed, however, a lasting tolerance to people passing by. In the early days Andrew would always hit a member of staff when they passed by. These improvements prepared the ground for the transition into adult services.

Andrew became much easier to manage in large group situations which previously he had found over-stimulating. We started (May 1997) the transition period to the social services day centre which he would attend upon leaving us. We commenced weekly visits, primarily for lunch. From day one Andrew was exhilarated by the company to such a degree that in the over-excitement Ann and I were subject to a constant flow of pinches – proximity around the lunch table adding to Andrew's advantage.

Other clients approached to say hello – naturally quite anxiety provoking for us. Andrew was pleased with this and these encounters rarely ended in a pinch. In an aim to integrate Andrew into the service, one client was put forward as a special friend. Andrew did respond to this, however – the 'old man' within couldn't resist and he availed himself of an opportunity of a passing hit on Margaret's back.

Recognising the achievement

Andrew didn't have to change, he could have stayed the same or got worse. The prospects for Andrew before our project, on becoming a client of a social services establishment (if a placement could have been found) would have been to sit in some corner of a unit deeply engaged in self-stimulatory activities – perhaps with staff in fear of coming near. Change was based on a combination of contributory factors which are now outlined.

A therapeutic approach to behaviour management

The strategies that we devised evolved through an understanding of autism and a knowledge of Andrew as an individual. Our timing seemed correct in that we planned no major interventions until we felt we understood him sufficiently, and a relationship based on trust and valuing him as an individual had evolved (establishing for him that he had something to offer the world and should not be viewed solely in terms of his behaviour).

Defusing skills were designed to bring calmness in high arousal, comfort and reassurance in anxiety times, order in times of confusion and resistance to intimidating tactics by Andrew seeking to dominate his environment. We became skilful at early identification of likely problems by being sensitive to the environment and to slight changes in Andrew's behaviour as possible forerunners to behaviour disturbance. Good and effective communication and trust developed between us. All action was carried through calmly, confidently (outwardly at least) and purposefully. Our performance was low key to allow Andrew as much opportunity as possible to self-regulate.

Our staff team had no ego problems – we were not tempted by a tough 'we'll sort him out' approach, which is sometimes heard of even in these enlightened times, and which we think would have contributed to Andrew becoming even less socially available. The performance by our little team was born out of a real desire to serve, a positive attitude towards Andrew, 'hands-on' learning, and aided by the provision of relevant courses which truly accelerated our professional development, sometimes inspiring new ideas and sometimes confirming our direction. Personal reading was also of benefit.

We received enough feedback from our recordings and Andrew's visible attainments to suggest our behaviour management strategies worked. We realised also, that the criteria for success needs to be measured especially on how well Andrew managed situations which were challenging for him. Total avoidance of potentially difficult situations was not a realistic policy.

The development of a therapeutic environment and curriculum

As a supporting system to our behaviour management policy we continued to address anxiety by developing a balanced curriculum in that stress-inducing situations were counterbalanced with soothing ones. To this end we built a pleasing environment in which to work and in which activities were included: walks on the Downs, the use of the Snoozelen room, listening to soothing music.

This proved to be extremely beneficial in terms of stress reduction. Secondary advantages arose from this, for instance, communicative exchanges with other walkers. In the context of the Snoezelen room, initial massage was met with resistance and at times a torrent of blows. Eventually though Andrew would routinely ask for 'more' with his own strategy, developed for the occasion by holding out his foot. Other advantages evolved from these practices. To use the example of the Snoezelen room, Andrew began to track the movement of projected visual images, initially he had insufficient interest even to look. His listening skills improved, for example, we were listening to classical music, and when the tape stopped Andrew attempted to turn it over.

Communication needs were effectively targeted (within the limitations of the time available)

During the course of the project Andrew achieved a greater comprehension of communication, and an increased ability to communicate. This was effected by our performance in making communication more accessible to him, teaching new skills and, above all, motivating him to engage in the act of reciprocal communication. As a result, much routine frustration and anxiety for Andrew were reduced. A great deal of work still needs to be done on communication, particularly the means of expressing emotional states. Our work had involved making him more aware of his emotional condition, i.e. telling him how he was feeling, and also taking preventative measures to reduce upset, such as keeping him well informed.

Summary

Andrew made a conscious choice to grasp his new lifestyle – he couldn't wait for the taxi to come for him in the morning. In doing so, he responded to staff directives, and learnt new skills. His communication became more frequent and of a more positive nature. Improvements in relating to other people grew simultaneously and were equally impressive.

Andrew's level of personal happiness rose substantially, he gained more control over his life, and his awareness of the world and other people in it was heightened. He became less fearful, of entering into new activities and experiences in case they held unpleasant consequences for him. His tolerances grew, as did his motivation to please others.

Andrew will always be a difficult person to be with and will require a high level of support throughout the rest of his life. With the correct provision he will achieve some degree of personal happiness within the limitations of his disabilities and a degree of control over his own life.

He continues to do well at the day centre and is now joining in more activities there. His expectation of encounters with other people continues to be positive – perhaps the most valuable achievement of the project is the development of his will to relate to others. He also continues to enjoy the experiences of coffee shops and walking, thanks to the efforts of the new staff who were like-minded to our philosophy in this area. His experience of life has been extended. Apparently he has a liking for ten pin bowling.

As for Ann and I, personal satisfaction was paramount as well as gains in experience and understanding. Stresses were great, at times more from outside pressures than Andrew himself: no premises initially, constant insecurity of tenure at Chestnut, an ongoing debate about extending Andrew's time in education, the initial rushed nature of the day-centre placement, to mention but a few. But we all came through and Ann and I would repeat the experience again.

Acknowledgements

We are indebted to support from colleagues at Hazel Court School, notably Peter, Louise and Pippa who laboured greatly on our behalf, Andrew's key worker Tony, and other staff at Chestnut Drive, and members of the intensive support team, Roger Noble and Sandy Ramdas, who all added to the success of the project and to making it a more memorable and pleasurable experience.

References

Jordan, R. and Powell, S. (1995) *Understanding and Teaching Children with Autism*. London: John Wiley.
Mesibov, G. B., Schopler E. and Hearsey, K. (1988) 'Structured teaching', in Schloper, E.

and Mesibov, G. B. (eds). *Assessment and Treatment of Behavior Problems in Autism.* New York: Plenum Press.

Watson, L., Lord, C., Schaffer, B., Schopler, E. (1989) *Teaching Spontaneous Communication to Autistic and Developmentally Handicapped Children.* Austin, TX: Pro-Ed Inc.

Zarkowska, E. and Clements, J. (1994) *Problem Behaviour and People with Severe Learning Disabilities: The STAR Approach.* London: Chapman and Hall.

Chapter 9

Commentary: managing incidents of challenging behaviour – practices

Dave Hewett

Introduction

This chapter gives advice on some basic practicalities of a working style that is brought about by application of the principles outlined in Chapter 6. It focuses on the tactical thinking and the personal style for members of staff who operate those principles – the detail of what they can actually do in challenging situations, issues such as what to say, when to say it, how to say it, where to stand or sit, and how to stand or sit. Once again it must be stressed that the material of this chapter is a general guide. It is still necessary to think creatively and apply the advice to the multifarious situations that may be encountered. There is a great emphasis here on thinking, making judgements and working from principles.

This style is part of an ethos where challenging behaviour is basically seen as a communication of inner state, where the person with the learning difficulty is not viewed as totally and solely responsible for their behaviour and progress with it, where staff seek to understand and work with the service user rather than simply banish the undesirable behaviour. This ethos places an emphasis on carrying out focused work with the person at times other than during the incidents of challenging behaviour, and coping well with the incidents when they arise.

A word here about physical restraint – use of overpowering physical force. One of the functions of the practices set out here is to give regard to everything it is possible to do in order to make physical restraint an absolute last resort. That is the clear orientation too of all of the contributors to this book. Actually, it is difficult to find a practitioner who openly disagrees with this attitude. It is the case, however, that many staff may not have the techniques, nor perhaps the will to make it a reality.

There will not be advice on carrying out physical restraint. That would be the content of a whole book in itself, and I actually do not consider it the sort of learning that should be conveyed in a book. It is my view that physical restraint is rarely necessary. There is no doubt that some people's behaviour is such that it is necessitated, no matter how good one's incident management, and when that is the case it must be done well. My concern, however, is that too many staff receive training in physical restraint, without correspondingly intensive training in the attitudes, techniques and creative thinking which go with making it an absolute last resort. The best courses on physical restraint cover both topics.

The advice set out here is aimed at assisting with thinking about getting the most out of the best tool one has – you, a person – face, voice and body. The work of the contributors is littered with examples of insights connected with the practitioners' awarenesses of how they were using themselves and their presence in order to seek to be effective with the person whose behaviour they were attempting to manage.

People who are members of staff working with people with learning difficulties may not give enough attention to how powerful they can be with simple communicative behaviours. Many may attempt to be powerful with complicated, 'powerful-seeming' behaviours. The practical techniques set out here are actually not difficult to have or to acquire, but they can seem that way. It is very much more difficult to employ these techniques if the first principle of being calm and having ordered behaviour is not attended to. It is also difficult when working with colleagues dedicated to attitudes of punishment and 'not letting people get away with things'. Being under extreme stress to get incidents of challenging behaviour over more quickly than is realistic can also be a barrier to acquiring these techniques.

Good managers of incidents of challenging behaviour are good communicators. In such situations, good communicators operate from good principles and give appropriate regard to the use of personal style to be effective. Good communicators also give maximum regard to the effects of their personal style on the person being challenging, so that as effectiveness starts to be achieved, it is recognised.

The stages of an incident

A helpful tool for thought and action during incidents of challenging behaviour is given in Figure 9.1. This was originally drawn up by Arnett (1989) and can be seen in Arnett and Hewett (1994) and Harris and Hewett (1996). Its first intention was to help with thinking around the more serious incidents of violence and aggression, but it works well for thinking at all sorts of levels. It has been modified slightly for the purposes of this chapter. In Chapter 5, this graph was referred to as a pre-prepared 'mental structure' which can be carried in the memory and help staff work through a person's incident of challenging behaviour.

The graph plots the progress of a person's arousal. Arousal has already been discussed as escalating feelings such as anger, frustration, distress, anxiety, fear and so on. The very worst moments of violence and destructiveness are likely to occur near or at the peak, the 'crisis' point. However, a person's behaviour is likely to become more difficult the higher they go up the arousal line. On the other hand, some people are likely to be quite difficult to be with while still at the lower stages of arousal.

The graph shows very smooth lines going up and coming down. This is an easy way of thinking about and remembering the graph, but the reality is that arousal often builds in a more untidy way as shown in Figure 9.2. However, many people may seem to have an extremely short reaction time from triggering to crisis, and

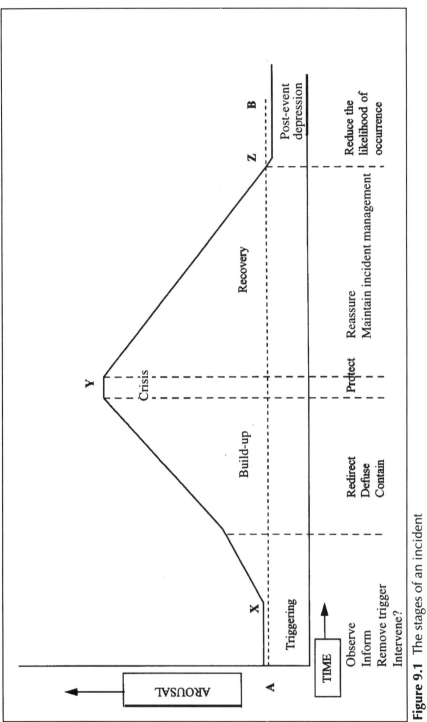

Figure 9.1 The stages of an incident

A. Arnett (1988)

we would conceptualise their lines as smooth and short.

The escalation and de-escalation is shown in terms of five stages: triggering, build-up, crisis, recovery, post-event depression. These stages are notional, a helpful device for using the graph as a mental tool. In reality of course, it is difficult to have any precision about where one stage ends and another begins. Additionally, there is no particular time-frame to the sequence. Some people go from triggering to crisis in three seconds, others may take three days.

Note that throughout the discussion of this graph of an incident, the model does not apply only to the person being challenging. It can also apply to the member of staff. Feelings such as anger and frustration can be triggered by a service user's behaviour. This can result in the scenario that by the time the person with the challenging behaviour is nearing crisis point, the member of staff can be well into the build-up stage. This is more likely to occur if the staff are not putting appropriate work and thought into preparation and into remaining calm and ordered.

Another way of looking at the graph is to view it as something entirely natural. It is a schematic representation of something that nature and evolution has equipped human beings with for good reason. It is a way of representing that familiar phrase concerning human defence mechanisms, 'flight or fight'. Sophisticated and mature as a society may be in the way that it is organised, our culture and our laws, the reality is that physiologically, human beings are probably little different from the cave dweller of 50,000 years ago. When presented with certain stimuli – danger, things which would make one frightened or otherwise aroused – the cave-person had the luxury of a more simple response than our society may advocate. The cave-person would probably get ready to fight tenaciously or run away very fast. Evolution had been very helpful and equipped humans with a physiological mechanism to go with the stimulation. Chemical-producing centres in the body are also triggered by this stimulation and

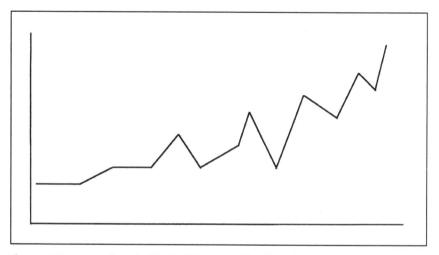

Figure 9.2 Arousal probably builds more like this

chemicals such as adrenalin are released. These chemicals do various things: they get into the muscles and charge them up, so that the cave-person fights better or runs away faster; and they get into the brain – if you are going to fight well or run away fast, it may not be helpful to be reasonable nor rational, so the chemicals help you to become more unreasonable and irrational the higher one goes into arousal.

This is, of course, a simplified scenario, but this sort of effect is probably happening to the person whose behaviour one is managing. The person becomes less reasonable and rational the higher the arousal. Awareness of these effects is crucial to the 'tuning-in' needed to make judgements about what state of arousal the person has got to, and, accordingly, what action to take.

The triggering stage

In Figure 9.1 the dotted line A–B represents a person's normal arousal. 'Normal' arousal is an elastic concept, occurring when a person is not experiencing feelings such as frustration, anger, fear and so on, and when body systems are at an everyday optimum. Most people experience a normal state of arousal when they are quiet, conversing quietly, walking along the street without worries, watching television perhaps (though the advertisers put a lot of thought into manipulating human arousal while watching television).

Different people's state of normal arousal may be at different levels, indeed some people with challenging behaviours may have a level of arousal which is normally very high. Many people with learning difficulties may experience, due to their difficulties with understanding what is going on around them, ongoing anxiety as a quite normal arousal state. Some of the contributors to this book write about service-users they are working with where this seems to be the case. Additionally, normal arousal probably goes up and down somewhat, it is given as a straight line for the benefit of the simplicity of the graph.

The trigger is shown as an event occurring at point X. Trigger is a word in fairly common use in work with people with learning difficulties and challenging behaviour. Most staff I meet associate with use of the term, both linguistically as a meaningful concept, and in practical terms because they see it happen.

I think it is important and helpful to dwell briefly on the meaning of the word as it is being used here. The trigger is the event occurring either within the environment or within the person which activates the state where the person's behaviour becomes challenging.

Examples of triggers within the person are:

- thoughts;
- memories;
- pain or discomfort;
- hunger;
- thirst.

Around the person triggers can be:

- noise;
- other people's outbursts or aspects of their behaviour;
- being shouted at;
- being goal-blocked;
- being too hot, too cold, etc.

Triggers can be many different things for different people. Of course, there is a sense where an external trigger is also an internal one, since it triggers some processes inside the person, but this contributes to the perception of behaviour having its source in a complex of factors. Figure 9.1. contains advice for staff action during the stages.

Observe
Observing, seeing things happening and knowing what you are looking at seems a rather obvious aspect of staff technique. However, it can be an elusive skill and one which may need further work and discussion by individual staff and teams.

However, the first indications of triggering in a person should lead to staff surveillance and vigilance – this should be the start of 'tuning-in'. Members of staff need to start monitoring the person for the signs and signals that the person's feelings and behaviour are starting to escalate, or are de-escalating. These signs and signals can vary greatly between people. The staff working with Trevor (Chapter 2) show good awareness of signals from Trevor, and how varied they can be:

> Trevor's entry into the classroom often gives me plenty of clues about how he is feeling that day; how he opens the door (tentatively or pushed strongly on its hinges), how fast he moves to his seat, the quality of his noise making, whether he gives eye contact . . . sometimes he sways gently and moves his hands rhythmically, other times he sits very still. Tuning-in to Trevor takes time and needs active discussion with other staff in handovers, core groups and team days to get the message across. It is hard. Yet there is no firm rule. He can be tense and quiet, also tense and noisy. Sometimes he gives lots of eye contact but this can mean he is in a more heightened state than if he shifts his gaze uneasily. (Pam Grounds, Chapter 2)

The list in Figure 9.3 attempts to illustrate this diversity. Some individuals, such as Trevor, may have several different ways of behaving which indicate triggering. The list is also intended to illustrate that it is difficult to have hard and fast rules which apply to all people. As Pam Grounds shows, it is partly a matter of getting to know the person and, crucially, sharing that information in a group of staff.

Staff should also look for the effects of the triggered person on the other people present. Are other people being triggered? Are other people the trigger, and can an intervention be made to reduce the triggering effect? Have other staff also observed that a person is in escalating arousal? These moments will be the start of

- obvious general change to more robust, noisy behaviour
- becoming more still and quiet
- increased rate and intensity of self-involvement, e.g. rocking
- the production of certain stock, learnt phrases, 'don't you dare!'
- increased eye contact
- reluctance to make eye contact
- eyes widening
- a certain vocalisation which is only produced during escalating arousal
- attempting to move away from other people
- body language 'stiffens'
- facial expressions 'stiffening'
- going red in the face
- going white in the face
- obvious attempts at physical self-control, e.g. clasping hands
- laughter
- voice 'tightens'

Figure 9.3 List to illustrate the variety of signs from people which give information about triggering and escalating arousal

the thinking and anticipation which will inform quick judgements during the next few minutes.

Inform

If other staff do not seem to be aware that a challenging incident may be arising, then they should be informed, sometimes with a simple word gesture and eye point if the staff are experienced at working and communicating with each other. These communications may also knowingly invoke the sensible procedures that staff working together have prepared for these situations.

Should anyone else be informed? There are some judgements to be made here about the other people with learning difficulties who may be present as part of a group. Whether to inform them about the likelihood of an impending incident may be influenced by their levels of understanding, and their likely reactions to the information. Certainly the judgement should be influenced by factors such as how much easier it might be to clear the room when necessary if everyone is prepared, how much better other people might cope with their own feelings if they are forewarned about an impending situation and, of course, how such a discussion will affect the person who is already triggered.

Remove the trigger

It is sometimes easy to be familiar with a person's triggers. The person may be routinely triggered into challenging behaviour by visible, regularly recurring external events. An obvious course of action then is to make sure that the trigger is not present in the person's environment, which is a sensible thing to do. In the account by Nicky Bond and Don O'Connor (Chapter 3) the staff fundamentally identified the way in which Andrew's challenging behaviour could be triggered by the behaviour of other people, sometimes by other people behaving quite normally. They accepted this reality as one of the bases of the way that the team worked, becoming particularly careful with their interaction styles with Andrew at all times. At the same time, they worked sensitively and over a long time to help Andrew to deal with his anxiety about the presence and behaviour of other people. They worked hard to help him become a better and more confident reader of what other people were doing and to reduce his general anxiety levels.

It is important to recognise that the trigger is not the cause of the person's behaviour. The cause is much more deeply rooted within the factors which contribute to the person having challenging behaviour. These factors are likely to be a wide variety of things existing within the person and occurring around the person (see Chapter 1). It can feel for staff that when they remove the trigger, the cause of the person's behaviour has gone away, because the challenging behaviour is no longer present. However, the factors, especially the personal, internal ones which have contributed to the person providing incidents of challenging behaviour, are still there. Personal factors particularly need some detailed, understanding work from staff. Personal factors may include things such as a lack of self-esteem, high anxiety and difficulties with communication. In the philosophy and outlook of this book, it is not the only intention of the practices advocated to make the challenging behaviours go away.

However, it may be decided that, as far as possible, known environmental triggers are removed from or avoided in a particular service-users' environment. On the other hand, this decision may not be made for various reasons, such as the staff undertaking a controlled project of assisting a person to cope with the presence of the trigger. This issue is dealt with in detail by Zarkowska and Clements (1988). Generally it is certainly good judgement, as far as is possible, to remove an identified trigger once the person has progressed well into build-up. The continuing presence of the trigger is likely to continue to contribute to escalating arousal through the 'build-up' stage.

Of course, it may not be possible to remove an external trigger from the presence of a person, or it may be an unknown internal trigger. In these circumstances, judgements about intervention need to be made.

Intervene during the triggering stage?
This decision can be very difficult. 'Nipping it in the bud' can and should be one of the tactics available to staff, and is more likely to be used by staff for people known to escalate to the more serious type of behaviour at crisis. In such circumstances a procedure may well be prepared for early intervention. Some other considerations may come to bear on these judgements, however.

Many people, even those with the more severe learning difficulties, have probably developed some abilities to cope with their own arousal. They may have learnt to defuse themselves by having experienced being triggered, going into build-up, but nevertheless being able to bring themselves down again with little or no assistance. This learning is highly desirable. As offered in Chapter 1, helping service-users to learn approaches to self-coping and to self-control are aspects of the framework of helping them 'learn how to behave'. Naturally, the point to be considered here is that this experience and the learning which may accompany it can be denied to a person if interventions are routinely made at the earliest stages of their escalation to challenging behaviour. So, difficult judgements may need to be made. Here are some suggestions to assist with the thinking:

- Don't have intervention at the earliest possible stage as an absolute rule of procedure. Make different judgements about interventions for each individual.
- Try to develop the confidence to stand back and keep observing. Observe particularly sensitively for signs that the person is coping well without help.
- Even if an intervention is still ultimately necessary, evaluate positively for the good work that the person carried out unassisted and use that information during the next situation.
- If it is felt necessary to intervene regularly as soon as possible, work hard to develop those interventions to be the minimum necessary for effectiveness. Monitor this process, do record keeping on it. Experiment also with the timing of an early intervention, perhaps gradually leaving it longer before intervening.
- If a service-user is showing signs of coping better with her/his own triggering, don't forget to let her/him know that you saw it, and offer congratulations. This decision will be tempered by knowledge of the person's communication ability, but some positive feedback should be possible.

The build-up stage

During this stage one has moved on from considerations of the triggering stage and is now definitely dealing with an incident of challenging behaviour. Even at the lower stages of build-up the person's behaviour is likely to be noticeable and significant, prompting decisions about interventions. Deciding which intervention to employ will be based on knowledge of the person from previous incidents and from information gleaned from moment-by-moment tuning-in to the person's signals. Remember that no matter how routinely similar this person's incidents usually are, and no matter how effective the agreed procedures, one should stay alive to the possibility that this incident may be completely different. People can be like that.

Some people's incidents never reach an absolute crisis point. They may become triggered and go into the build-up stage, but perhaps stay for some time at a higher level of arousal where their behaviour is definably challenging, but perhaps with 'ups' and 'downs', as shown in Figure 9.4.

Redirect

Redirecting a person can only occur at lower levels of build-up, where the person's arousal levels are still not so high that a state has been reached where reason and rationality are no longer available. Again, individual judgements need to be made; depending on ability and understanding, together with other aspects of emotional make-up. Some people are not amenable to reason and rationality even at apparently low levels of arousal.

Redirecting implies calling a person to order, looking for co-operation, and even being directive about doing this. In the process of being directive, it is important that while being assertive, perhaps authoritative, the personal style used is none the less not too dissimilar from the defusing style of the next section and that one's style does not contribute to a growing and needless conflict. This may mean making direct and authoritative statements, but at the same time ensuring that facial expression, body language and tone of voice remain reasonable and respectful, and especially that sounding aggressive or intimidating is avoided. These things *can* be combined with a sense of authority.

There are two particular reasons for this care in style. Firstly, this style is likely to be more successful with more people in achieving acceptance and agreement to redirection. Secondly, if the person continues to escalate into levels of arousal near crisis point, it is harder for the member of staff to switch style completely into being a defuser. It may be harder because there is a feeling of 'climb-down' from a previously highly authoritarian style which demanded compliance. It may also be more difficult for the person being challenging to respond to the change of style in the member of staff. The contributors show examples of staff making clear 'boundary' statements to the person they are attempting to manage while not contravening an overall communicative and defusing style. Actually, I for one, despite my not inconsiderable physical stature, have always been next-to-useless at getting people to do what I wanted by giving them stern, authoritative orders.

Most staff who operate this style effectively talk about their reluctance to shout

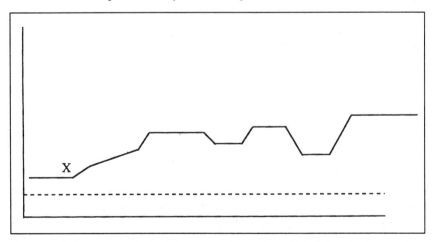

Figure 9.4 Some people build up to a plateaux at a high level of arousal

or even raise their voice over-much. Bernie Hunt and Peter Brooks (Chapter 6) illustrate this as an extreme embargo on this use of voice, even while working with the potentially most difficult people of all. The contributors to this book all seem to favour use of voice which may be direct at times, but is also conversational, using the tone with an expectation of co-operation and participation rather than a demand for absolute compliance. It can be natural sometimes to use a questioning style:

'Oh, come-on, let's get up yeah?'
'Alright then, do you want to sit down now?'
'Come on, come over here with me.'
'No, you know you can't have that now don't you?'

Use of directives phrased as questions can be helpful and may indeed help people being challenging to co-operate, since they are not being presented with a direct order or ultimatum, which it may be tempting to challenge further. An order or ultimatum can lead to the member of staff escalating the situation, since the ultimatum may bring with it a sense of absolute enforcement. Avoiding direct orders or ultimatums can help the member of staff to keep trying and working with the person. As mentioned, it is harder to switch from absolute enforcement into a defusing style if the situation keeps on escalating. Additionally, if re-directions are well phrased to avoid ultimatums, the member of staff can eventually give up if necessary. This occasional necessity is not to be sneezed at. Some residential staff I worked with were having difficulty getting a resident out of bed to go to the day centre. They had put a great deal of work into their style in the mornings, learning the hard way to avoid giving rigid orders and ultimatums, since in the end there was nothing they could do if the person absolutely refused. It was not a situation which warranted resort to physical force. They felt also that giving rigid orders actually heightened the resident's sense of triumph when they 'lost'. Of course, this issue is fundamentally related to staff outlook, particularly the values associated with whether service-users have the right to say 'no' and the extent to which staff have the duty to persist (see the discussion in Chapter 1).

Some staff groups I have met hold the view that they should not be using the questioning style at all, since the person does not have a choice, she/he is expected to do what they are told (this applies particularly, but not only, to some educational establishments). I feel that they are missing out on the use of a valuable technique, and are more likely to have confrontations with this value 'carved into stone'. Additionally, it is a quite normal aspect of communication in our culture to phrase requests or even orders in this way. I do not feel that people with learning difficulties should be excluded from this.

'Delayed compliance' is another technique sometimes seen. Actually, since the word co-operation is preferred, perhaps it should be 'delayed co-operation'. This is a redirection which can apply to situations where leaving the situation briefly will be possible, as with the residential establishment mentioned earlier. It is simply to do with the member of staff making the point, 'Come on, time to get up now', but if necessary leaving the person with the proposition, 'alright, I'll come back and ask you again in a few minutes'. The interval might allow the service-user to cool somewhat and be more amenable on the staff member's return. It can be repeated if necessary. It can be taken further and a different member of staff be sent the next time. It just might have been the first member of staff who was the problem that morning. Staff can only operate like this, however, if they are not fixed on compliance, if they have communal team values, and if they have a sense of realism about their position as authority figures.

Another frequently overlooked aspect of the use of redirection is remembering to positively reward the person for having been successfully directed. A few generous words at that moment are likely to have a fundamental effect on the success of the next such intervention. Burchess (1991) stresses this issue by giving redirection techniques the full title of 'redirect–reward'.

Defuse

Defusing techniques merit detailed discussion in a dedicated section, following this description of the stages of the graph. These techniques and skills are the fundamentals of incident management, in that while defusing tends to be a set of things to be attempted with people who have reached the build-up stage, knowledge and experience with them tends to affect a member of staff's style of working at all times. A skilled defuser becomes a member of staff who may well exhibit more calm assurance generally. The skills may become so integrated into an overall personal style that incidents of challenging behaviour seem to happen less around that member of staff. As has been mentioned, there are some lucky people who seem to have natural abilities with being calm themselves and with dealing with other people's behaviour in apparently 'charismatic' ways. These things, this personal 'atmosphere' can be learned. Reassuringly, even skilled defusers sometimes get it wrong, have a bad day when everything blows up, or they do not necessarily even have the expectation that they will get it right every time.

Contain

As build-up increases in the person being challenging and probably in the general atmosphere, it is important to try to contain what is taking place. It would be foolish for a team of staff not to have agreed and even rehearsed procedures for this if it is a regularly recurring similar incident. Containment is concerned with doing everything practical to minimise the effects of the challenging behaviour, examples include:

- making sure the person being challenging has got enough physical space;
- other service-users may need to be distanced from the person either by moving the person being challenging if that is possible or by moving the others if that is possible;
- the availability of another space for either of the above eventualities;
- having enough staff present for managing all this. Is it possible to get more?;
- making sure that any favoured or likely weapons, missiles and so on are removed;

- identifying and reducing all potential environmental stresses, e.g. music, other noise, too many people;
- and, of course, having incident management practices concerned with defusing the incident.

The list above is only some of the things which need to be thought through. Most of them are really rather obvious and perhaps do not need to be listed as aspects of staff technique. However, part of the intent here is that there is nothing too basic or obvious which cannot be thought about. One small staff team I met wrote a procedure for the next likely incident with a man who had threatened with a sharp knife. The procedure was good and sensible in all respects except that it did not include removing sharp knives from the kitchen during the triggering stage. Another team refused to move the other service-users from the presence of a person who was liable to throw furniture. They held the view that if the person being challenging would not be moved, they did not see why other people should be 'inconvenienced'.

Thinking these things through quickly in the heat of the situation can be difficult. This invokes once again the need for staff to do everything possible to achieve calmness in their practices.

The crisis stage

Not all incidents of challenging behaviour are ones where the person being challenging escalates to an absolute crisis. Many service-users may provide quite exciting and challenging incidents without hitting a true crisis point. The crisis is viewed as those moments of violence, of destructiveness, of an extreme outpouring of behaviour. The crisis point is shown on the graph as being brief, perhaps just a matter of seconds. The expression of feelings at this point is intense and it would be rare indeed for a person to stay at crisis for a long time. However, it may feel as though some people provide a prolonged crisis. It is more constructive and helpful perhaps to view their crises with a modification to the graph, as in Figure 9.5.

This graph pictures the person having a sequence of crises in quick succession. The first crisis is followed by a small dip out of crisis, but some triggering agents are still present for the person. Very often these may be inner triggers such as thoughts or feelings. Even after having just had a crisis, the person is still at a very high level of arousal, and therefore all the more sensitive to being re-triggered, so another crisis is the result. Naturally this is very difficult for staff to deal with, and we might describe this scenario as the very worst kind of incident.

On the other hand, this view of what is taking place can be helpful because it may cause staff to think about any things happening in the environment which are triggering the person back into crisis: the original trigger to the incident may still be present, or it may be some other environmental event. I once got punched (hard) because I leaned into the vicinity of a person's face to tell him off in

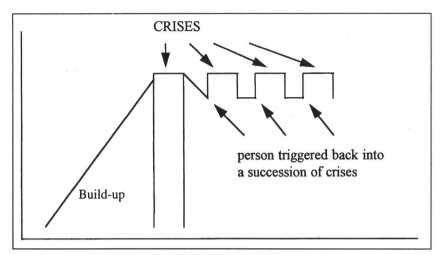

CRISES

person triggered back into
a succession of crises

Build-up

Figure 9.5 Modifications of the 'stages of an incident graph' – a person
who seems to have prolonged crises

'gritted-teeth' style for having just broken a window. I have seen numerous
people who have just thrown things, be told immediately to 'go and pick it up!'
Making recompense for something 'bad' you have just done may in some
circumstances be an appropriate way of bringing the 'badness' of the incident to
the person's attention. However, it is important not to have an absolute rule for
this and to make judgements about the person's level of arousal. It feels foolish if
the person goes and picks up the object, but immediately throws it again.

Protect

It is difficult to give firm advice about possible interventions during the crisis
stage except to say that the best protection advice is for staff to do everything
possible not to intervene. If the person's crisis has the nature of ranting, leaping
around expressively, rocking furiously, tearing clothes, destructiveness that is not
too hazardous, then it may well be that the best judgement is to use the defusing
technique 'do nothing', followed by doing as little as possible as the crisis passes.
The work of the staff at Womaston House illustrates these judgements (Chapter
2).

It can be very tempting for staff to do all sorts of things immediately after the
person's crisis has seemed to pass. Service-users may behave in many different
ways immediately after their crisis outburst. At one extreme, some will have still
extravagant, but gradually diminishing displays of behaviour. Other people may
become immediately still and quiet. It can be especially tempting to start
admonishing the ones who become still and quiet. The upper levels of the graph
are shown in Figure 9.6 as a means of remembering that although the absolute
crisis has passed, the person is still likely to be at a high level of arousal and care
must be taken. This is especially true for the most serious incidents, but the
principle applies to people whose incidents may not be so daunting nor hazardous.

163

Wait and reassure

This is where staff really demonstrate their ability to deal with their own feelings. It is understandable that staff can feel upset and even outraged by people's behaviour, particularly for instance, if someone vulnerable has been hurt. Staff who are maintaining their calm are in better shape to operate the priority concerning avoiding an immediate re-occurence. The best practice, as shown in Figure 9.6, is to avoid doing things which may impede the person's progress downwards from crisis. This may mean doing very little to or with the person, giving both physical and psychological space, but staying 'tuned-in' and maintaining all protection measures for everyone else. It is worth holding on to the attitude that the incident may be over in terms of the extremes of behaviour, but it is actually still the recovery stage for the person – we are still in incident management. With some people, it might be judged necessary to keep a member of staff nearby offering calming (see 'defusing', this chapter). Judgements here may be influenced by the effectiveness of calming immediately before the crisis.

'Reassurance' is a key word, and anything that is done to or near the person while in recovery should use it. It can be difficult to feel reassuring toward someone who is the offender. The contributors all offer help on this. They illustrate that the value system that they bring to their work – caring, having compassion, not holding people solely responsible for their feelings and behaviour, avoiding blaming – can translate into moment-by-moment practices such as holding back their own feelings and behaviours and being positive with the 'offender' at times such as these.

The post-incident depression/aftermath stage

The graph shows that some people may not only return to normal arousal after an incident, they may dip below it and experience a type of depression. Not all

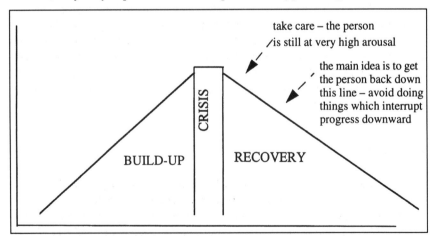

Figure 9.6 The upper levels of the 'stages of an incident graph'

people do this, some return to their normal selves more quickly and are once again available for all the usual activities.

What should be done during this stage is once again concerned with judgements made on an individual basis for each service-user. Some people who experience the 'depression' may need to be simply left. Others, during a depression, may actually be more emotionally available, more inclined to an emotional and psychological reconciliation. The theme is to make judgements about what will be most effective for each person and to do things which contribute to a reduction of the 'likelihood of occurrence'.

Bernie Hunt (Chapter 6) looks for debriefs with the person, judging when she/he is once again rationally 'available'. If the service-user has the ability to take part in verbal dialogue, the debrief might be on a continuum from, 'Okay we've done something wrong. Something has upset you I know', to 'Look that really upset me and other people in the classroom. Where did that come from?' If the theme of the debrief is to request the service-user to exercise more self-control in future, this needs to be placed within the context of the person's ability to do this and to understand the requirement.

On the other hand, in their work with Trevor, the staff seem more orientated toward the priority of making available a long period during which Trevor gets back to normal. This long period, together with recognition of Trevor's communication abilities, makes a direct, analytical debrief with him less of a priority. This perspective seems to be shared by Rosemary Hawkins (Chapter 11) and Bernard Emblem and staff (Chapter 4). Their concept of the 'aftermath' stage is all of the rest of the time that the person is not being challenging. Their pupil's abilities are such that doing any detailed debriefs or perhaps using 'blaming' are not feasible. The emphasis is on getting the incident over effectively and quickly, and having the person back in good shape to carry on working on communicating, relating, developing a growing sense of order, structure, reason and control in their behaviour. They rest their incident management practices on the same understandings of the pupils that drive all of their other work with them.

Several of the contributors to this book emphasise their recognition of the need for staff to debrief. This may be emotional support, emotional unloading, making sure they do a technical evaluation, doing whatever is necessary to put them back into a position where they can deal with a similar situation. These needs of staff are very frequently overlooked or the hurly-burly of the working day doesn't seem to allow for them.

Defusing

The higher a person goes on the arousal line and the less likely it is that she/he will effectively manage her/his own behaviour, the greater should be the tendency for staff to commence defusing. There are various defusing techniques, some of which will work only if there is still access to the person with dialogue. At the very high stages of arousal, the defuser is likely only to be 'calming'.

Two words can be found in common usage to describe the processes – 'defusing' and 'diffusing'. They are often used interchangeably. 'Defusing' gives the image of taking the fuse out of the situation, 'diffusing' the image of dissipating it, spreading it widely. Either word is meaningful to describe the activity, 'defuse' is the one preferred here.

Defusing requires giving maximum attention to the person who is being challenging. It requires the member of staff to be thoughtfully operating the principles outlined in Chapter 5. It is particularly important that the defuser is focused on no other priority than achieving an effective outcome – incident over, everything calmed down, nothing broken, nobody hurt. Other considerations such as blaming, punishing, telling-off and giving therapy can all wait – this is not the time for them. They can be dealt with when the person's arousal state has returned to more normal levels. A classic mistake is for staff to use telling off – 'not letting him get away with it' tactics – when the person is at a very high level of arousal.

As has been stressed, a good defuser is a member of staff who has sufficient calmness and internal order to think clearly and tactically. The most basic technique is 'calming' – it is the only technique to be employed when the person has crossed the line E–F on the graph (see Figure 9.7 for a further modification to the 'stages of an incident' graph), However, the staff personal style which goes with 'calming' should be the basis for all defusing techniques – modified and elaborated upon, but running as a consistent 'thread' in the staff style.

There are a few basic categories of defuser:

- calming;
- de-triggering;
- distracting;
- response to reasonable need;
- do nothing.

They can be used in combination, modified and refined as aspects of the style of individual members of staff. Their use may also be refined and modified as an outcome of experience with an individual service-user. Each will be enlarged upon in turn.

Calming

The skills involved in using calming are beguilingly simple – it can be difficult to be good at calming. On the other hand, once regular acquaintance with the skills is achieved, there is a tendency to wonder why other methods of attempting to manage a person were ever preferred.

Calming is the ability to use your own behaviour and interaction skills to assist an angry, frightened or otherwise aroused person to de-escalate. The emphasis is on communicating willingness to help and reassure, even offering to assume 'control' by helping the person to become more calm, together with the message, 'You need not fear me'.

The intention to 'do the least to achieve the most' is a guiding light in calming.

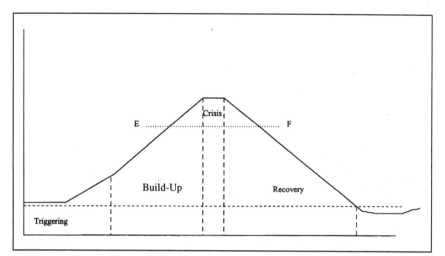

Figure 9.7 Modification of graph showing the E-F line

The behaviours employed by the member of staff should be simple, predictable and reassuring. The only intentions of calming are to prevent the person from escalating further in arousal or to bring the person down to a level below the E–F line. Other defusing techniques which might involve dialogue or more complex behaviours, can then be employed. The E–F line has been added to the graph to indicate a notional stage of the person's arousal, where her/his state is such that she/he has entered the 'danger' zone. Above the E–F line the person is likely to be somewhere beyond reason and rationality, will probably neither hear nor understand speech very well, will have become ultrasensitive to other people's behaviour, will need little more to happen in the immediate environment to push her/him into crisis. I believe I have met many people with learning difficulties whose difficulties with the world are such that they live most of their daily existence on or near an E–F line.

A person who is calmer gives maximum regard to using simple communicative behaviours. In this way a member of staff can become immensely powerful and effective in incident management by attending to these matters. Some guidelines to each of these things are given here, but it is important to remember that these are good general guidelines. They are not absolute prescriptions for staff activity, which take away the need for staff to think and use good judgement.

Voice

Any statements should be made briefly, should be concerned with reassurance and the transmission of calm and be repetitive if necessary. Voice should be kept even and relatively low in volume. It is better to resist temptations to talk over the top of the person or to use a louder voice. Any bombardment of the person with speech should be completely avoided, it is far better to say little and/or to repeat simple statements such as:

'Okay . . . okay.'
'It's alright Mike . . . alright.'
'Come on . . . that's fine'
'Yeah, that's it . . . take it easy now.'

Deliberate use of pauses after any statement is good technique. This gives time for the effect of the use of voice to sink-in with the person being challenging, it enables the member of staff to avoid speech bombardment and also gives time to 'read ' the person being challenging and think about the next action. In this way all use of voice should be measured and controlled, with the member of staff assessing continuously for positive or negative effects on the person.

Face

The things happening in the member of staff's face should parallel the use of voice. Facial expression should be steady, even, not changing too much. A person at this stage of arousal does usually feel immensely powerful, whatever other emotions, such as fear, are being experienced. Their sense of power should be accepted and their desire for attention respected. Therefore, facial expression should also show clearly that attention is being given.

Eye contact requires care, but on the whole good, steady, communicative eye contact should be offered or maintained, and is potentially significant and effective. Staff need to be able to recognise if the other person is objecting to eye contact because it feels threatening or too intense for her/him at that moment. Some people actually mention this, 'Stop looking at me like that!' If signals of discomfort with eye contact are received, it should be removed immediately. It is not necessary to look completely away, lowering gaze to the person's knees is usually sufficient and enables a member of staff still to 'read' the person's body language and facial expression with peripheral vision.

Smiling should be avoided. Use of humour can be a good defuser, but very rarely at this high stage of arousal. Positive, reassuring smiles as the person is being successfully defused and coming down might well be useful, but probably not above the E–F line.

Body language

Body language is more difficult to describe. Movements should be smooth, deliberate, slow, even and radiate a sensation of control and poise, even when it is necessary to move quickly. It is easy to ask people to relax their bodies, but very difficult to do unless a member of staff is experienced or a natural. None the less, the best calmers will have relaxed neck, shoulders and arms, hands open and visible, weight distributed to one side in a relaxed posture when standing. Hands can be used carefully in those relaxed 'calming' movements that can be a very natural communication, and they may then also be in a good position for protection if necessary. A summary of all these aspects of staff style is given in Figure 9.8.

It is easy to include some don'ts:

- don't fold arms;
- don't place hands on hips or hitch thumbs in belts or pockets;

- don't do the 'gunfighter' – feet well apart, weight evenly spread (one of my old favourites actually);
- don't wave hands and arms around;
- don't clasp hands behind the back;
- don't point or use a raised finger;

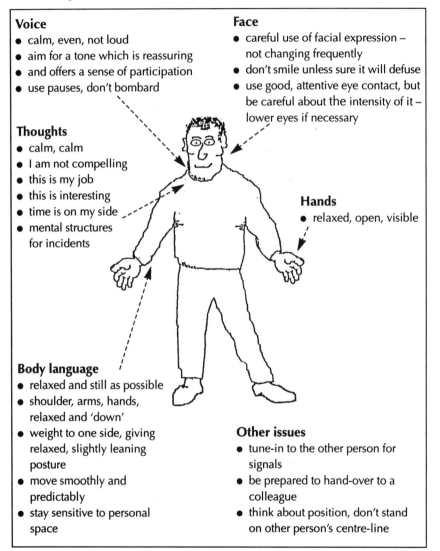

Voice
- calm, even, not loud
- aim for a tone which is reassuring
- and offers a sense of participation
- use pauses, don't bombard

Thoughts
- calm, calm
- I am not compelling
- this is my job
- this is interesting
- time is on my side
- mental structures for incidents

Face
- careful use of facial expression – not changing frequently
- don't smile unless sure it will defuse
- use good, attentive eye contact, but be careful about the intensity of it – lower eyes if necessary

Hands
- relaxed, open, visible

Body language
- relaxed and still as possible
- shoulder, arms, hands, relaxed and 'down'
- weight to one side, giving relaxed, slightly leaning posture
- move smoothly and predictably
- stay sensitive to personal space

Other issues
- tune-in to the other person for signals
- be prepared to hand-over to a colleague
- think about position, don't stand on other person's centre-line

Figure 9.8 The Defusing Style: Being a calmer. The calming style for the most extreme incidents or an incident near the crisis stage is illustrated. As the person comes down from that level, this style can be gradually modified and elaborated upon, with the member of staff starting to do and say more. This style of staff behaviour should also form the calm basis for use of other defusing techniques, however.

- don't clench fists;
- don't jig about or sway from side to side;
- don't lean forward.

Sitting or crouching can be employed, especially if the person being challenging is sitting. Many people with learning difficulties whose crises are likely to be less serious in terms of what takes place, may be sitting in a chair or on the floor, or even lying. Staff should make a judgement about sitting, however. Sitting down or crouching can give good non-threatening, reassuring body language, but may also render a member of staff more vulnerable and less able to move away quickly. Getting into a sitting position can also be a complex set of movements, so care with the deportment is needed.

Positioning

A calmer or defuser's use of positioning can be critical. The obvious general rule is not to get too close. Normal personal space is likely to be an arm's length away or just over. A person's sense of personal space tends to grow with arousal and she/he is likely to be more sensitive about the boundaries of it. Figures 9.9 and 9.10 illustrate some principles of the use of space and position. Firstly, in terms of space, it is better to be further away from the person than too close. Several paces away is a good minimum, but this is also one of the areas where the member of staff should be tuning-in for feedback information from the person as to whether one is too close. If a member of staff is 'reading' the other person well, it may be possible to keep a good space, but move closer and use the voice more as the person becomes more calm.

A basic principle of positioning is illustrated by use of the dotted line which runs straight out from the person being challenging: don't stand on that line, stand to one side of it.

When people wish to be aggressive and challenging to one another, if they are building-up to a fight for instance, they tend to stand on the centre line of each other's position, so that they are absolutely square-on, shoulders parallel, face to face. In this position it is much easier for the conflict to escalate. There are psychological effects such as feeling compelled to sustain rigid, challenging eye contact, and a deep feeling that one's escape route is blocked by the other person. The closer to each other that people stand with this position, the greater the effects. Actually of course, this is also the classic position for telling-off a child.

A person being a calmer works much more effectively by standing one step off the line, with a slightly angled position relative to the other person, at a comfortable distance and with relaxed body language. This stance makes it much easier to transmit the non-verbal message: 'I am not threatening you or in competition with you, but I am here, I do want to cope with this situation with you, I am competent'. This message is the powerful sense of helpful physical presence that a good calmer will attempt to achieve.

The corresponding situation for when the person being challenging is sitting down is shown in Figure 9.11. The member of staff is giving regard to proximity and to staying off the centre line, but has crouched into a relaxed position beneficial to effective communication. In fact in this situation it is possible for the member of staff to have an eye-line which is lower than the person sitting. This can be enormously beneficial in helping to allay any message of confrontation,

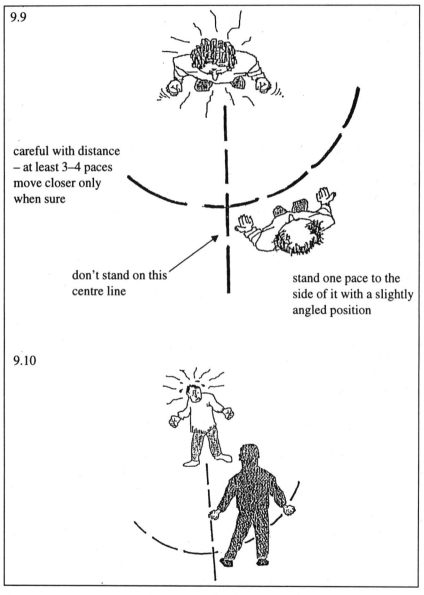

Figure 9.9 Positioning and proximity from above

Figure 9.10 Positioning and proximity from behind the member of staff

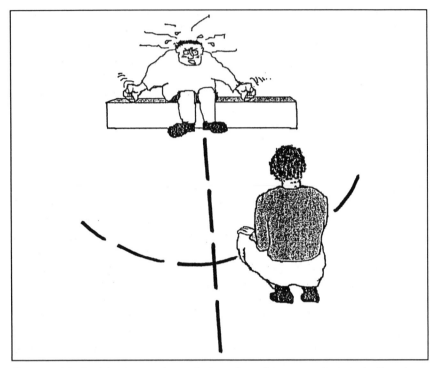

Figure 9.11 Positioning and proximity when the person being challenging is near crisis and seated

while not affecting the message 'I am here, I am competent'.

There are exceptions to these principles of positioning. Even people at quite high levels of arousal may respond to being approached by a good calmer, being given soothing physical contact even, particularly if this becomes a positive routine. This may especially be the case for people who are pre-verbal, where staff use positive physical contact routinely as an aspect of communication with the person. It is important that these aspects of defusing are not disregarded. However, the advice of the principles here is: move closer and enter personal space tuned-in and with caution – remembering the centre line as a principle of approach; use judgement about use of physical contact; move slowly and smoothly.

De-triggering

This technique is concerned with addressing the triggering factors in the person's arousal. If you know the triggers for the person on this occasion, it is as well to remove them, or to do what you can to minimise their impact while you bring the person's arousal down. Often, simply removing the trigger will be sufficient to defuse the person or to cease an escalation.

Additionally, de-triggering may be about discussing the triggers with the person and offering help with their effects, 'Alright, I'll come and help you look for it, yes?' Lewis Janes and his team (Chapter 10) routinely used this as a first-step technique. Addressing these issues can only be done when the person is at lower levels of build-up, certainly below the E–F line, and probably lower than that. At higher levels of build-up, the only issue is the arousal and it is probably a good judgement not to mention the trigger.

Distracting

Distracting is the technique of helping the person to think about something else other than the arousal. A distractor will be any option you can offer which will be a viable alternative to the arousal for that individual (e.g. a drink, a walk, an activity, a sit down, a talk, a quiet place, go somewhere different). Once again, decisions need to be made about what stage the person's arousal has reached. At higher stages it becomes less and less viable to indulge in the dialogue necessary to offer distractors.

Distracting is about alternative options, but also about giving the person power. Distracting makes sure that the person always has an option open which will enable her/him to decide to change the situation. Use of this technique contributes to avoidance of the win–lose scenario style of confrontation. A person who is powerless, with no options open, is more likely to choose to gain power by use of powerful challenging behaviours.

Care is needed. The distracting options chosen should be reasonable, practical ones which will not in themselves make things worse for the member of staff. All options should be as respectful to the person as anything done at any other time. Also, the person should not be bombarded with options, as this could aggravate them further. Distractors should also be offered, not insisted upon.

Response to reasonable need

It is always possible that staff may take the punitive view that an aroused person's 'anti-social' behaviour means that they forfeit all rights to receiving things until their behaviour has improved. However, it is good technique to respond reasonably if a person in build-up requests something that can be resonantly given. This 'response to reasonable need' can be treated as a distractor. Staff can use their sense of calm presence and movement and take a little time to supply this need, with the person hopefully watching and waiting. Once again, cautions about what is 'reasonable' for both the staff and the person being challenging apply.

Do nothing

This is an often-used technique used intuitively by many parents, teachers and staff of all descriptions. Bernard Emblem (Chapter 4) describes its use with some wonderment at the sense of serenity the staff were showing. Its absolute basis is the reality that a person who goes into build-up, *will* come down again, eventually, even without assistance. The problem is that the consequences in the meantime may force judgements about making an intervention. This is why the technique when used, must be used with good tactical judgement that the consequences of not intervening will be manageable.

At the extreme, many staff everywhere have experience of, in the end, having to stand back and wait while a person 'blows'. One (very large) person I worked with could frequently be defused, but staff also recognised a threshold in his signals where the technique was something like: 'Okay, we haven't done it this time, clear the room'. He would then indulge in five minutes or so of therapeutic furniture-throwing, with staff monitoring constantly from a safe distance. Naturally one of the things to be monitored for, one of the judgements is: will he harm himself in his rage? If the answer was yes or maybe, some further and probably hazardous interventions must be considered.

On the other hand, the use of pause in staff defusing behaviour has already been discussed. The member of staff doing nothing at tactically opportune moments can also be viewed as a thread running through good defusing technique. In fact, the good defuser will probably spend more time doing nothing other than radiating calm presence, than she/he will in contriving to do 'something'. A member of staff I met who was fed-up with the frenzied activity of colleagues in difficult situations had a good motto: 'Don't just do something, stand there'. Good, tactical use of doing nothing is a significant aspect of the principle of staff avoiding contributing to the seriousness of the incident with their behaviour. It is good technique and a good calming agent, to be prepared to do nothing at judicious moments during incidents. In particular, when staff find themselves in that awful situation of not knowing what to do next, doing nothing and having a think for a few seconds (whenever possible) is probably better than doing something ill-judged.

References

Arnett, A. (1989) *Dealing with Violence*. Hertfordshire Social Services Training Department Course materials.

Arnett, A. and Hewett, D. (1994) 'Safety First', *Community Care*, 10th March.

Burchess, I. (1991) *Who Needs Help with Challenging Behaviour?* Kidderminster: BIMH.

Harris, J. and Hewett, D. (1996) *Positive Approaches to Challenging Behaviour.* Kidderminster: First Draft Publications.

Zarkowska, E. and Clements, J. (1988) *Problem Behaviour in People with Severe Learning Disabilities: A Practical Guide to a Constructional Approach*. London: Croom Helm.

Chapter 10

Leading a well-challenged social services residential team

Lewis Janes

Introduction

In January 1996 I took up the post of team leader at a home in Chard for people with severe learning disabilities and challenging behaviour. I was a newly qualified social worker with ten years experience of residential child care covering three counties. I had considered all of my past experience to have been highly enjoyable until the six months before starting my training. The change in my ability to enjoy my work had focused around many changes in the 'Observation and Assessment' centre that I had worked in. These changes created a situation where verbal and physical abuse directed towards staff members was a daily occurrence. This negative experience had a massive effect upon my confidence in working with children, so I had made it very clear that I wanted to focus on another client group during my training. The resident group I had chosen was people with learning disabilities. I entered into this experience with an open mind, grateful to be doing anything other than child care. This open-mindedness was in fact naivety which often showed in my practice! However, I began to recognise that I could find more satisfaction working with these people than I had done for many years in child care. My two years training, although a difficult time for me as a student did, however, identify channels of work I was happy to pursue.

The interview I attended for the post was actually a joint interview for two posts. I had been keen on the other post which was for a new home for people who were much more independent and had not been 'labelled' as challenging. At interview I was keen to gain this post as I did not want to be 'labelled' as someone who only worked with 'challenging' people. I had endured my fair share of physical intervention and felt that I had an equal amount of skills in caring for rather than controlling people. This again perhaps demonstrated my naivety concerning the type of work I was going into.

I started work having spent a few hours, weeks before, discussing the job with the deputy, Pete. He described each resident and his perceptions of them and their life at the home and the work over the last few years. Clearly there had been many problems concerning the way things had gone and the staff team had endured an extremely stressful time during which their need for increased support had not been fully met.

The home had been set up a part of the county's response to the Community Care Act. Four of the original five residents had all lived for large parts of their lives in long-stay hospitals. Many of the behaviours I was therefore witnessing were classic repertories of learnt behaviours from such institutional care: the residents would rarely communicate with each other; they would often only communicate with staff to identify their primary needs; even this communication was greatly impaired as (for instance) they would have had little or no choice about what they would be eating or drinking or, indeed, what time they would be eating or drinking. Many of the residents had developed skills that did not relate to other skills they had developmentally. This seemed to stem from teaching plans that had identified day-to-day skills (e.g. making a cup of tea) that probably had little relevance to the actual opportunities available to the individual (the kitchen was always locked!).

The resident group had a vast range of disabilities and seemed in many ways not to be a compatible group. The home was in an advanced state of refurbishment and building which had gone massively over deadline, due to the inherent problems of agencies with different perspectives on priority having to jointly co-ordinate such works. This had lead to a situation where the five residents had to live in a four bedroom bungalow for several months rather than the promised weeks! The living and working conditions were unbelievably chaotic. This was evident in the behaviours that the resident group were manifesting. There were many incidents involving self-harm, anxiety, aggression, confusion and chaos. The staff team had managed this situation well considering the chaos. Much of the management had focused on medical intervention which struck me as not being appropriate. This point was going to be an area that was easy to focus on. I had worked with many children who had demonstrated similar levels of distress and we had never considered the use of medical intervention. This was an important factor in my beliefs about the way forward. Clearly it represented the different philosophies of 'medical model' versus 'social model' mirroring the history of children being brought up in care homes and adults being locked up in hospitals. One enormous difference in this approach was that the children I had worked with could tell me what was wrong or how they felt. These adults had no speech but they were still communicating very clearly, often through the behaviours labelled as challenging.

Some of the resident's day-care needs were being met at a local day-care resource centre. There seemed to be regular conflict with our residents and the other 'more able' residents and staff at the centre. I felt that many of these conflicts were direct communication from our residents that they did not want to be there.

Brenda

Brenda was one of the residents that seemed to regularly be involved in 'challenging' incidents at the centre and had seemed to have developed quite a formidable reputation. This reputation had evolved during a lifetime of 'institutionalised care' – clearly the recognition (or lack of it) of Brenda's autism had played a large part in her life.

Until the age of three, Brenda had presented as a 'normal' happy child, if somewhat independent. Brenda's mother began to be concerned about her development and had taken her to the GP. Significantly, her mother had watched a TV programme about autism just prior to the GP visit and when the doctor asked what she felt was wrong with Brenda she suggested autism. Brenda's mother is able to talk freely about the lack of understanding and support regarding autism during this time. What I find most remarkable about this is that Brenda's mother is now able to be so supportive to us as a team considering the 'poor deal' she has faced from the 'professionals' in the past. Brenda was placed at age 7 in a school for the deaf in Devon. This placement – though it did begin to develop Brenda's skills in communication through sign – was not successful, and the picture of challenges began to develop. From there Brenda went to a large hospital for the 'mentally handicapped'. Here she was able to develop many skills, both practical and social, but again the developing pattern of challenges was evident. This was almost entirely managed through medication (not unusual considering the constraints upon staffing levels within such institutions). It was during this time in the hospital that Brenda was formally diagnosed as being autistic. When the hospital was in the process of closing as part of the county's response to the Community Care Act, Brenda was one of a group of people who were the last to leave because of their identified complex and challenging needs.

Pete had described Brenda to me as 'autistic'. This was already a very keen interest area for me (as I had worked closely with a man with Asperger's syndrome during my training and had gained such a valuable insight into autism from him because he was able to discuss how it affected him in many aspects of his life). So I looked forward to this work. Considering the confusion of five people living in such a small area with such differing needs it was obvious that life could not be very enjoyable for Brenda during these changes. Pete was quite open about his frustration at the staff team's inability to understand autism or even accept that Brenda was autistic, often describing Brenda as difficult or unpredictable. At this stage I was not aware that there had been a diagnosis of autism, so I felt it was important for the team's understanding of the complex problems they were facing.

This was an area that I felt needed to be addressed. A formal diagnosis was given describing some of the behaviours Brenda was presenting as typical of a person with autism. The staff team still did not respond markedly to this. It was at this stage that I began to understand how important training regarding the specific issues and understanding of autism was going to be. Actually, while writing this 15 months later, I none the less still question how successful this aim has been and to what extent we have succeeded in getting life right from Brenda's point of view.

In her file, Brenda's person description was as follows:

Physical description: Brenda is about 5'4" and of slim build. Her hair is fair and very curly. Her top teeth are slightly protruding, her nose is wide and she has several raised scars on her forehead. She also has piercing blue eyes.

Brenda has an ungainly walk that looks like she is limping.

Brenda is a lady with severe learning difficulties and behavioural problems. She is deaf and has great difficulty in communicating, although she does understand some total communication, she is not good at signing back.

Brenda has very obsessive behaviour which may lead to her self harming or hitting out at staff and residents, e.g. she has her own special puzzles and if any parts of these gets mislaid Brenda will turn the house upside down looking for the missing puzzles. While doing this she will bite herself and bang her head, she will also hit out at staff, and can quite seriously injure by scratching, head butting and biting.

Brenda can also be very unpredictable while travelling in a vehicle, especially when on a road that she is not familiar with, if she does 'blow' she will go for other passengers and the driver.

Brenda needs to be watched at all times as she can be so unpredictable, laughing one minute and hitting out the next. She also gets very upset with herself and others if she cannot convey what she wants, this also leads to the behaviour mentioned above.

NEVER TRY TO HANDLE BRENDA ALONE, CALL FOR ASSISTANCE.

I was more than shocked at reading this description. Without having met Brenda first I think I would assume that she should carry a 'Government Health Warning' around with her! Having read this material, it is also worth noting that this description had not been updated since May 1993.

There had been significant incidents involving Brenda over the years, these had lead to staff being injured and often property being damaged, particularly cars. I can therefore relate in some ways to this person description. However, it did convey an incredibly negative image of Brenda and did not attempt to identify the skills she did have. She had a good understanding of signs and would use them. If these signs were not interpreted accurately enough by the staff members then she would get anxious and angry, possibly resulting in self-harm or lashing out at the staff member.

The method of communication developed in Somerset is called Somerset Total Communication (see also Chapter 7). It has been developed by the speech therapy department as a way of supporting a people with a great range of communication difficulties. The method involves using hand signs, prompts such as pictures and photographs, as well as speech. This method was successful with Brenda, but the staff team often did not seem confident in using it. This was another area that caused me frustration, in many ways my own inexperience was beneficial in this area. During my training I had been involved in observing a number of speech therapy assessments. This gave me an insight into just how easy it is for staff working with people with learning disabilities to aim their communication either well above or well below the other person's ability by making assumptions about what they perceive the individual to be understanding. This experience has made me realise just how important it is to support our speech with prompts such as signs during our communication with even the most able learning disabled people.

My 'induction' – thinking further about Brenda

I chose to spend the first two weeks observing the resident group and how the staff team supported them. I cannot remember a day during that time without a headache. How the staff team had survived several months was a miracle. The resident group of five consisted of four men aged between 24 and 49 and one woman, Brenda, then aged 28.

One resident spent up to 23 hours a day chanting, yelping, jumping and spinning. He would also take any food or drink he could see (whoever it belonged to). Another resident spent much of his time trying to get into the kitchen to drink tea. If this need was not met he would head bang on the floor to such an extent that he had created massive injuries to his forehead. Another resident seemed quite happy, always chatting (often repetitive words); however, he would bite his own forearm when distressed. Another resident spent much of his time pulling down curtains and pinching things that did not belong to him.

All these behaviours contributed to the impossibly chaotic life that clearly was not healthy for a person with autism because many of the residents would be creating changes such as moving or damaging objects without Brenda being there to see and therefore understand the changes. The designed move back to the main house for Brenda would obviously be a much more conducive environment because she would have much more of her own space and the other residents in the house tended to have a greater understanding of other people's privacy and space. At this point it is worth noting that I make no apologies for using the term autistic – yes, I am perhaps 'labelling' a person and this does go against much of my training. My beliefs are that this label is in fact an incredibly strong tool that will enable a higher level of understanding for those working with autistic people. It will not necessarily enable empathy – the confusing difficulties with life that can confront Brenda and others can be literally incomprehensible for the rest of us. However, by giving people a greater understanding of autism we are enabling them to accept the behaviours more.

(There is always an ongoing struggle in reinforcing this new understanding when staff members have experienced traumatic incidents that necessitate objective thought, following events that can be interpreted very personally. Yes, that's easy for me to say if I'm not the one who has just been punched or scratched!)

This belief also represents my identified aim in providing effective training to enable the whole team to develop a framework of understanding and then meeting Brenda's needs as a person with autism.

During my observations of the first two weeks it seemed that the staff team had developed a method of working with Brenda (during her episodes of anxiety or agitation) that was quite successful. The incidents seemed to invariably focus around Brenda searching for something and getting more and more agitated as the search progressed without finding the missing object. The working method seemed to involve supporting the search in the 'communal' areas, but blocking any attempts Brenda would make at searching in other people's rooms. It is worth noting that other people's rooms at this stage included the kitchen!

The guidelines were written up as 'strategies that may work when dealing with Brenda':.

1. Diversion: e.g. puzzles, different environment, different activity, such as making a drink.
2. Medication – chloropromazine, up to 20 ml.
3. Total communication and interaction with Brenda. Let her try to solve the problem herself. Do not allow Brenda to direct you physically, i.e. grabbing staff.
4. Non-threatening. Do not crowd her. One member of staff to deal with Brenda, one member of staff to support.
5. Look for signs of Brenda's distress. Try to identify what might be causing Brenda's distress, e.g. something missing or moved.
6. If Brenda becomes either a danger to herself or to others, remove her immediately and briskly to a quieter environment.
7. Give Brenda the attention she needs, but do not allow her to manipulate the situation. Brenda needs to know what her boundaries are.
8. Brenda needs continuity and consistency.
9. If nothing else works, use your physical intervention training, as a last resort.

The above written work clearly contained many practice areas that are important when dealing with difficult situations. However, the sequencing of the methods may have inadvertently led to the issues being avoided, particularly point 2 – medication. This is an area that would need to be considered much later in an incident. There is also quite a high level of control during the incidents, rather than giving Brenda the control, e.g. point 3, do not allow Brenda to direct you physically. Because Brenda has no speech her 'directing' of staff was quite a sophisticated method of communication which needed to be developed rather than avoided. Often this 'directing' would be seen as aggression because if the staff member did not respond then Brenda's grabbing would become more insistent and could lead to scratches being given.

While acknowledging the 'scary' nature of some of the incidents, it is worth pointing out that some responses during episodes that scare can directly increase the negative behaviours. One point in particular seemed to be that when some staff felt that they were nearing the stage when a punch might be aimed at them they understandably started to face away from Brenda. This unfortunately cut off a massive proportion of the communication Brenda was potentially receiving.

The following points are important in considering the working method:

1. It was a home for five people that at this point only contained four bedrooms. One of the residents would regularly take other resident's belongings.
2. While I was able to understand the staff team strength of purpose in trying to prevent Brenda searching in other people's rooms, this did not take into

account any understanding of how Brenda's autism meant that she had to find the missing object. Often the fact that something had gone missing from Brenda's room was because a resident had already invaded her privacy and taken something from her room.

3. There were (at that time) genuine reasons why the kitchen was regularly locked, including a very limited understanding of the dangers of electricity, heat, boiling water, etc, by two of the residents. There were also reasons that were not valid for preventing people having access to the kitchen. These reasons had developed to the extent that the door to the squash cupboard was also locked because Brenda 'would always drink neat squash and then get aggressive when the squash was finished' or 'she gets demanding if there is no squash left.'

If the methods above were still unsuccessful the working method would then change quite dramatically. People would stand in her way, more staff members would become involved and doors would be locked.

This would lead to a rapid escalation of Brenda's challenging behaviours. She would bite her hand and bang her head against the walls with increasing strength. The next steps could include the opening of doors to bang her head on the edge of the opened doors. During these stages of anxiety she would also often strike out at staff members with a clenched fist. Once the 'extreme' levels of self-harm were evident then a medication of chlorpromazine as required (PRN) would be administered.

Being able to look at incidents objectively it seemed clear that the initial approach being used had merits. Brenda would be supported in her search and communication would be encouraged (clearly a mutually beneficial experience). However, when the staff involved felt that the search had been exhausted they rapidly made a decision (without involving Brenda) and the approach changed direction, rapidly becoming aversive (locking and blocking!).

Clearly there is a great dilemma around the issue of Brenda searching another person's room. Looking at it from Brenda's perspective there is no dilemma (she is looking for her own belongings in another room in her house). However this does challenge the 'philosophy of the home' and I understood the struggle staff members have with this. The only training we are able to give concerning this area was to reflect upon incidents that have already happened to enable the staff members to understand Brenda's reasoning for entering another person's room. The question of any possible impact on the person (whose room it is) also needs to be considered as well as their understanding of the situation. It could be argued that if the other person is not present then there is no impact, again this is an area that many (including myself) do not feel comfortable with, but as reflective practitioners our understanding of past events should enable us to come to terms with this dilemma.

Developing the approaches to Brenda's difficult behaviour

There was clearly scope for change in the way the team worked with Brenda, particularly around the team's understanding of:

- the way Brenda communicates her needs and anxieties;
- incidents of aggression (self harm and to others);
- the importance of some of the 'odd' rituals Brenda presented much of the time;
- the team's ability to reflect on some of the incidents and learn from them.

Everyone who has witnessed or been involved in difficult incidents such as those Brenda may present can understand just how disturbing and frightening they are. The feelings generated in us as staff can interfere with our own clear thinking about the tasks we face. A major task seemed to be to identify improvements in the management of behaviours while enabling Brenda to be more involved in her own management and reducing the team's controlling methods during the incidents.

The following points are worth considering:

- During these incidents Brenda is often communicating at quite a high level, often through sign, always by leading or pulling staff members to the site that is causing her concern, perhaps where she thinks the missing object is. The increasing strength of Brenda pulling a person's arm can be interpreted as a 'challenge'.
- Brenda is actively seeking the support of the staff members in her search.
- The use of medication is seen as successful! Brenda calms down. I can understand this approach, but I don't agree with it. Who receives the respite? Brenda or the staff members involved. It is also worth considering how, while the philosophy is working away from the 'medical model' it also reinforces it. For instance, staff above a certain scale can perform such tasks, but having a higher scale does seem to be a reward for gaining these skills. Why do we not give people pay rewards for receiving training on values and attitudes of working with challenges using communication rather than physical intervention?
- There was and still is to some extent a belief that sometimes Brenda is not actually searching for anything at all! The cop out clause! This reflects part of my ongoing work in encouraging staff to reflect upon and write up incidents in such detail that they can identify what Brenda is actually searching for and also just how much communication she is giving and receiving. Providing an environment where staff can identify incidents and look at them critically has been invaluable, concentrating particularly on areas that Brenda would have found difficult, such as changes that she has experienced but has found difficult to communicate.

The ongoing process of staff training aimed at enabling us to respond to Brenda with understanding about how her autism may affect her has been a focal point for much of my work over the last two years. The formal training has been two half-day sessions for the whole staff team. The first day was to identify basic principles behind autism, the triad of impairments. This was an opportunity for the training group to explain some of the current thinking regarding autism and to look at some of the behaviours people with autism often present. The second session was for the staff team to identify some of the work incidents they have experienced and then look at the incidents using the triad of impairments as a way of understanding how or why the incidents developed.

The informal and ongoing training has involved discussions during team meetings about incidents and behaviours, again trying to understand them using the triad as a framework of understanding. On the whole I have found this process very rewarding and quite revealing. It has also enabled me to often 'check' my assumptions about individual staff member's ability to understand what (I believe I now more fully understand) is an incredibly complex issue.

It has been useful to consider this training while looking at some of the incidents that have occurred during the last year. This has enabled many of the staff team to understand more fully that Brenda is in many ways very predictable and does communicate well rather than 'Brenda can be very unpredictable' and 'has great difficulty in communicating'. After some of the incidents I have given staff hastily written questions to answer regarding the specific issues within the incidents, how they handled it and if they felt that there was a significant build-up to the incident. This process I feel has been useful as part of the debriefing process and is something I feel would benefit from being more of a formal procedure following incidents in the future.

We now have a new 'method of approach' for Brenda when she is experiencing states of high agitation. This new title for the intervention during challenges has enabled the team to focus on all the residents of the home and create specific 'methods of approach' for each resident's challenges. It identifies the positive aspects of the individual and enables the resident to have a higher level of control. It recognises that medical intervention may be necessary but that there are several other 'strategies' that can be used first that may be more appropriate and that the staff group have the skills to use. I feel that this piece of work has been a useful tool in identifying the staff that are able to understand more fully the change in approach and should therefore have more of a lead role in the induction of new staff members. It has also been useful for challenging staff members who feel that the approach is not successful. There have been various occasions when looking in more detail into the management of an incident it has become clear that the 'method of approach' has clearly not been used and has identified quite clearly at which stage the management failed. This process is not a comfortable one for some people, and it has been useful to involve the other staff members that were supporting during the incident.

The following gives the new method of approach. This is followed by descriptions of some of the incidents that have occurred during the last year and how they have been managed.

21/4/97 METHOD OF APPROACH FOR BRENDA WHEN
EXPERIENCING STATES OF HIGH AGITATION

Brenda is a person with autism and has a severe learning disability, she also has a profound hearing loss.

Brenda communicates most effectively with staff who use Somerset Total Communication. This must be supported by speech (as a method of good practice).

If Brenda is anxious she will demonstrate this in any of the following stages:

- becoming vocal, – this will increase in volume;
- intense nose-picking;
- becoming red faced and forehead sweating;
- increased sweating;
- lips becoming blue;
- searching;
- mobility will become faster;
- hand biting;
- head banging;
- scratching others;
- physical aggression to staff members – open-handed strike;
- physical aggression to staff members or other residents – closed fist strike.

Many of the causes of Brenda's states of agitation can be attributed to the fact that she is a person with AUTISM. She finds it difficult to comprehend and accept change.

Try to find out if anything in Brenda's environment has recently changed. Brenda will often assist with this by leading you to the 'site' that is causing her concern. Where possible allow this to happen. Communicate with Brenda, reassure.

Communicate with your colleagues to find out if they know if anything has changed.

Try to get Brenda's eye contact.

Sign to Brenda. 'Where', 'What', 'Calm down', 'Good', 'Bad'. This not only helps her to show you where the problem is but also helps her to remain calm.

Try not to use methods such as locking doors, cupboards etc., this may only lead to an increase in the behaviour.

If Brenda starts to head bang or hand bite then try to distract her by placing some of her puzzles out on her bed and making her aware you have done this. The puzzles must be placed carefully so not to create more agitation by losing any pieces.

If the hand biting and head banging stage increases then prn medication can be used at the discretion of a senior member of staff.

Incident – Monday 23 February

Brenda and resident C were going to go shopping, walking to the local shops. This had been communicated to them well through total communication (T/C) signs and speech. Both residents understood this well and had gone to get their coats. Brenda came into the office, took me by the hand as if to lead me outside. I signed that I needed my coat and it was in my car. Brenda came with me, she may have thought that we were due to travel in the car, but she accepted it when we went back into the house.

I looked around the downstairs rooms to check that all the doors were locked. Brenda followed. In the kitchen I noticed that the toggle on Brenda's coat hood was hanging down on one side and not even showing the other side. I showed this to Brenda and tried to pull the toggle free. It seemed that the stitches holding the toggle in were too tight. I pulled a pair of scissors from the kitchen drawer and showed them to Brenda. She pulled my hand towards the toggle so I cut the stitching and pulled the toggle free.

Brenda spent about two minutes looking at the toggle and then pulled my hand towards it. She seemed to want me to push the toggle up inside the coat as it was before, I then spent about ten minutes showing Brenda all the possible places the toggle could be, including where it was before. Clearly Brenda was not accepting this, Kath then joined in this process and we signed 'It's broken' and 'Put it in the bin'. Brenda would not accept this and was becoming anxious, this manifested itself in Brenda's face becoming hot and sweaty and shifting from foot to foot. These are signs of a developing anxiety level that are well known for Brenda. Kath then got the sewing box and showed Brenda the needle and thread. Brenda pulled this towards the toggle. She wanted the hole stitched as it was before. This Kath did. While doing this we discussed how (if at all) Brenda was dealing with this situation and what would possibly happen next. Brenda was not in any extreme state of agitation yet (this would have manifested itself in hand biting and head banging).

Brenda did not seem to accept the newly sewn toggle opening but she did follow resident C outside to the car. This demonstrated that she was not so distressed as she could be diverted to other things. I did not feel it was appropriate to take the trip in the car considering Brenda's level of anxiety as she was still picking at the toggle. We chose to walk to the nearby shops to buy some things for lunch. Kath and C walked ahead and Brenda walked with me. She then ran towards Kath and C, took Kath s hand and tried to pull her back to the house. I caught up with them and signed to Brenda to come back to the house with me. She did this and the others were able to continue to the shops. I felt that this was appropriate considering Brenda's state of anxiety was not extreme. We went back into the kitchen and spent another ten minutes trying different positions for the toggle. Although she was clearly anxious about these events, Brenda was still able to communicate with me at a basic level. We were both seated, facing each other in close proximity, as her level of anxiety rose she would stand up which made it more difficult for me to fiddle with the toggle so I would sign for her to 'sit down' and she would.

This episode had now lasted an hour and no progress had been made. I was aware that although her level of anxiety was not extreme (as she was not yet hand biting) this level was not far off, because of this I know that working closely to Brenda's head was potentially quite risky, as she could lash out at me. I felt I had no option but to carry on. Brenda then got up and ran to the office, she still had a good level of self-control as she signed to me 'key', rather than banging her head on the door, we opened the door and went it. Nothing in there to help! She then went through to the bungalow, presenting the offending toggle to Jan, our domestic assistant. Jan started work with Brenda, signing 'calm down' and showing great interest in the toggle; as this went on another member of staff came in with another resident, they had been out for a walk, and also Kath returned with C. Jan was still working with Brenda, trying different positions for the toggle and then (almost as if someone had flicked a switch) Brenda turned away, walked back to the house and went upstairs. We did not follow, hoping that Brenda might have gone to put the puzzles out (this is something she often does to calm herself down). Brenda walked back down to the lounge about five minutes later, she had taken her coat off and put it away.

The whole episode had lasted about an hour and a half, and eventually Brenda had accepted that the toggle was not going to look the same as it had done before. Although this was a difficult episode that effectively prevented the planned activity of a trip out from happening, I felt that it had been handled by all involved very effectively. All staff members had used T/C with Brenda. Brenda had been allowed to set the pace and we had not forcibly prevented her from looking for help from other people, we had not used any medication, although we had been able to discuss it as an option should Brenda's level of agitation have risen further. The communication between staff members during this episode had acted as support.

This whole episode again demonstrated a change in the staff members practice in dealing with Brenda's 'challenges'. We had used our skills, such as effective communication, T/C, predicting stages, understanding the importance of this issue for Brenda, communication between staff members during the whole episode and valuing Brenda enough to invest our time. This enabled her to understand and deal with the situation in her time not ours, rather than using medication or keys to lock things away.

Incident – Friday 24th January

Background

Brenda had been on several successful trips home to see her mother 30 miles away. We were confident of the success of the visits as long as Brenda clearly understood where she was going. We managed this by developing a system whereby Brenda would be given a letter in both symbols and words inviting her to her mother's house for lunch. We would support this through sign. Brenda would often respond to this by signing 'bus', 'home' and 'mother'. The only difficulties we had faced during these trips home were if we had missed any turnings, this would rapidly lead to Brenda becoming anxious, biting her hand and head butting the car windows. The trips home were developing in stages to allow Brenda's mother to spend time with her without staff members impacting on the household.

One significant stage had been where three staff members went with Brenda, one was left in the house with Brenda and her mother while Pete and myself left in the bus to go shopping. We had support for Brenda and her mother in the form of a staff member remaining in the house and a mobile phone in the bus to call us back should Brenda become anxious. This event had to be carefully planned by trying to explain through sign that we would be shopping then returning to pick Brenda up. It took several attempts with Brenda following and guiding us back to the house before we managed to get away without causing Brenda anxiety.

The next significant step was for Chris and myself to drive the bus with Brenda and another resident to Brenda's mother and then leave Brenda with her mother while Chris, myself and the other resident went for a walk and a pub lunch. This again took several attempts before Brenda was comfortable and understood that as the bus was staying outside her mother's house we would soon return.

Considering the success of the above trips I felt that the next step would be for Brenda to be taken by just myself to her mother's in my own car. The back-up to support me would be Pete and another staff member and resident following out of sight in the bus. Both Pete and myself had mobile phones so that if Brenda did become anxious and agitated then I would have support. I felt particularly confident in this plan as Brenda had been on several local trips with me in my car.

We approached the situation in the same routine with the letter to Brenda from her mother supported by staff members signing 'car', 'mother' and 'home'. Brenda happily got into the car with the letter and we set off. Brenda did show a few signs of anxiety during the first few miles and I was able to reassure her by showing the letter. We also stopped at a garage for Brenda to choose a chocolate bar.

Things were going well until my car came to a crunching halt with smoke pouring from underneath the bonnet. I signed to Brenda that the car was broken. She immediately showed signs of anxiety (biting her hand and punching the gear stick). I stayed with her in the car continually signing 'car broken'.

I was able to phone Pete on the mobile and he arrived with the other staff member and resident within five minutes. By then I had phoned the AA who were on their way. Brenda refused to get out of the car into the bus. She remained highly agitated, continuing to bite her hand, punch the gear stick and started to head butt the car windows. Throughout this, we all signed to her that the car was broken and we would drive to her mother's in the bus. Brenda did get out of the car briefly but quickly ran back and jumped in. I explained the situation to the AA man and he called for support from the police (so that the traffic could be slowed down). We quickly realised that this was a potentially serious incident considering the location (busy road) and Brenda's insistence on staying in the car. We called for further assistance from Paintmoor in the form of more staff support and some medication. This was clearly an incident that needed to be resolved by getting Brenda home as quickly and safely as possible.

During this time Brenda's mother was kept informed of what was happening. It was felt that a larger than normal dose of sedative medication was necessary to have a rapid and strong effect. Although I have these strong feelings about the use of medication, I felt that this occasion warranted its use.

The support and medication arrived and was given as Brenda continued to refuse to get out of the car. We continued to sign to her that the car was broken and that we had to get into the bus. One member of staff wrote in words and symbols on a piece of paper that the car was broken. This seemed to have been a significant factor in getting Brenda out of the car. The medication took 40 minutes before there were any significant reductions in Brenda's anxiety. When she did start to calm down she willingly got out of the car and into the bus which then quickly drove away, Brenda being given support in the back of the bus by three staff.

The significant factors within the reduction of the potential damage of this incident are many. There was a great deal of planning and preparation involved, not just in this trip but the ones beforehand. The staff involved were all confident and had a basic understanding of the specific needs of Brenda as an autistic person. In many ways this incident reinforced much of the training these staff members had received recently. The communication at all levels and stages was effective with all involved: Brenda, the other staff members, the AA man and the policeman. The last two people in particular needed quite a high level of reassurance to enable them to understand the situation.

The learning experience for me is that within the team we need to consider whether we need to take medication on the next planned visit. There was a still is a lot of planning towards such trips and in many ways this incident has highlighted just how extreme the potential dangers can be.

Incident – 5 February, 11.40 a.m.

Brenda entered the office and searched through the pile of papers on my desk. In the room were two visitors, Pete and myself. Brenda did not appear agitated and left the office. Two minutes later Brenda entered the office again, this time appearing a little anxious (red faced) again searching through the pile of papers, held my hand and pulled me towards the papers. I went through them. We could not find the things she was looking for. Brenda walked to the kitchen with Pete following. Pete and myself started to question what she was looking for and what stage of anxiety Brenda was now in. We felt that Brenda was looking for a book of shopping vouchers as there had been one in the kitchen and one in the pile in the office. Brenda led Pete up to a small pile of papers on the kitchen worktop and started searching through these. Pete remembered that he had cleared up and thrown away some papers from the night before. We both continually signed to Brenda that the book was broken and was in the bin.

We returned to the office with Brenda again and searched through the pile. She took me by the hand to the kitchen, looking for the other voucher book. We continued to sign that the book was broken and in the bin. Brenda was clearly beginning to get agitated (very red faced and sweat on her head). She was able to sign back to us as we signed 'where', 'look at me' and 'calm down'. Pete and I discussed where this incident was going, it was likely that the next step would be hand biting and then head banging. Pete remembered that the bin in the kitchen had not been emptied last night so he pulled the liner out and searched through it, quickly finding the voucher book. Brenda helped with this search and rapidly calmed as soon as the book was found. We again signed that the books were broken and had to go in the bin. Brenda was not accepting this and carried the bin liner (without the books) to the garage where the bins are stored. On her return she wanted to place the books back on the kitchen work surface. Pete took the books and encouraged Brenda to go to her room. She did this and then returned to the kitchen to make a drink of orange.

The significant factors within this piece of work are that Brenda was supported by two members of staff that she trusted. We both had a good underpinning knowledge of autism. We both could read the body language of Brenda's anxiety, we supported each other with questioning what Brenda was searching for. We supported Brenda by communicating with her through sign language. We respected her as a person by allowing her to have access to rooms and cupboards that she clearly wanted to search through. We were confident enough to work through her anxiety knowing the level and being able to predict the next steps. We were confident in the fact that we could use a prn as a last resort.

We were able to discuss this incident immediately after it occurred, which serves to reinforce our practice while acknowledging that such episodes can never be avoided.

Concluding thoughts

Developing the ability to reflect upon the practice concerning our work with Brenda during the last two years has been a valuable experience, informing our work with other clients as well as Brenda. The challenges we are now faced with are often similar to the ones that have previously developed so we haven't changed them fundamentally, but we do have less of them.

I am pleased with how effective the training programme has been, particularly around the change from the 'medical' model of intervention towards the 'social' model. This has enabled staff members to recognise just how skilful they are in recognising how the challenges develop and then supporting Brenda during them rather than controlling her. The training has always focused away from physical intervention, again another aim of mine. Ironically I feel that the next stages of this training process may necessitate some physical intervention training. This is because we have a new resident living in the house who (because of his limited understanding of the challenging incidents) often tries to get involved! This not only exacerbates the situation but places himself and the staff involved in an even more vulnerable situation. The senior team will need to consider carefully where we are heading with such training. Although I can foresee its need, my confidence in this area is significantly less than it has been during the other changes in practice.

We all have a greater understanding of Brenda as a person, but there is still scope for us all to learn more. I have found the changes particularly rewarding for a number of reasons, primarily because of the way Brenda now understands and interacts with her own life and the opportunities she has. Many of the team have grown as a result of this work, some have found it harder than others and have been able to look at their career directions as a result (this is not negative as they have been able to consider in a reflective manner the skills they have and look at areas where their skills can more suitably be used).

My style of management is now beginning to change. I can be less directive and this is particularly evident in the work we are doing with the other clients' challenges. Having set the background to the 'methods of approach' through guidelines, each co-ordinating group now creates their own for each client. For the team to be able to own this work has been very effective and again highlights the development that staff are able to look at situations in an objective manner and benefit from supporting each other through this.

Part of my change as a manager has also been that I recognise more fully where the team were 'coming from'. I have a greater understanding of just how stressful and frightening many of the incidents have been and still are. However, we have learnt to debrief objectively and to learn from this reflection rather than argue and blame.

Brenda's care and support is never going to be easy, her life as a person with autism will always be impacted by change. Not only will her care givers change (as all staff teams do) but the service as a whole will inevitably change. It would be naive to think that change can be avoided but it is worth recognising that change (even for Brenda) can be healthy, by providing new opportunities for Brenda to demonstrate the skills she has. Brenda's relationship with her mother continues to grow, the trips home with lessening support will continue (gearboxes permitting!). This will hopefully lead to Brenda going for overnight home visits with no staff support (still a long way off, but not impossible).

The role of medication within Brenda's life is now greatly reduced, and there is still scope for more change. However, I now recognise more fully that there are occasions where the challenges cannot be resolved without medical intervention. Having said this, the amount of prn medication needed continues to decline, evidence itself that the team are supporting and managing the challenges using the skills and knowledge they have developed. My understanding of the difficulties Brenda can present has in many ways changed during the last two years. However, what I have gained from this work is an insight into just how much fun she can be to work with and how rewarding seemingly small occasions, such as Brenda walking into the office, pointing to the safe, then the car keys and my jacket, because she wants a drive to the newsagents to buy a bar of chocolate. That is not an incredibly disabled person, it is a person with a disability who is incredibly able.

Chapter 11

Ann – the challenge of a difficult to reach five year old

Rosemary Hawkins

Introduction

As I looked down at the small tear-stained face, a big pair of hazel eyes, full of pain, gazed back at me, and for just a second, we met! In that moment I caught a brief glimpse of the anger, sorrow and deep frustration of this fellow human being.

I too had felt such pain, but unlike this child, I had been given words with which to express my feelings. She could only plead with her eyes, in the hope that someone, somewhere, might at least begin to understand and meet her in her pain. At that precise moment I began to dimly comprehend that my task was to be that 'someone, somewhere'.

My heart went out to this child, and I felt challenged to find ways to touch her, and children like her, at some deep level. This led me to begin the search for ways to develop communication with pupils with severe learning difficulties, in an attempt to give them a voice whereby they could share their inner-most thoughts, feelings and fears.

I remember the first time I met Ann, she was walking along a corridor holding a member of staff's hand. On the outside she was a very attractive five year old, full of life and bounding with energy. As I approached a sudden change descended and for no apparent reason she collapsed to the floor, crying uncontrollably, thrashing her arms and legs, and sobbing in absolute despair. When I asked the staff member the reason for this dramatic change, I was told that there seemed to be no reason and that this behaviour occurred at several times each day. A few weeks later, I became Ann's class teacher and discovered just how frequent and unpredictable Ann's mood swings could be. My first task was to get to know this child, so I decided to gather as much information I could about her in order to gain some insight. Here is what I discovered.

A profile of Ann

Ann was almost six years old, a strong, fully mobile child, full of life. She is the second eldest child of a family of four girls, three of whom have severe learning difficulties. She has an older sister, aged nine and two younger sisters aged four and two years. The four-year-old sister appears to be making normal developmental progress. Ann suffers from epilepsy and although on medication to control this, she still experiences seizures during the school day, which often leave her distressed, difficult and exhausted. Her statement identifies several special educational needs including the need to develop communication, awareness of her environment and to improve her self-help skills and independence.

When I joined the already established class group as their new teacher, Ann's behaviour was an overriding factor within the classroom. It was interfering with her ability to learn new skills, and was deeply affecting the total learning environment and all those working within it. Although Ann had no structured verbal communication, she did have the ability to be very vocal in a loud and intrusive manner, raising the volume within the classroom to an uncontrollable level! When staff attempted to pacify her and distract her with a variety of activities to channel her energy more purposefully, their success was negligible. Ann remained isolated and only calmed down when left free to roam around the room, very much on the edge of the group. Even this apparent peaceful mode was only temporary, for after just a few moments there would be another destructive outburst against the classroom equipment or displays or, worse, against herself.

Therefore there was an urgent and desperate need to find a way of intervening which would reduce this 'challenging behaviour', and replace it with a more communicative repertoire. So, in September 1995 when Ann moved into a new class group, the staff who worked with her decided that the management of her behaviour was to be given priority.

It was thought that a great deal of her inappropriate behaviour was perhaps due to her inability to communicate her wants and needs to those around her, and the frustration this must cause her. The staff felt that were they to provide new ways for her to express her desires, then perhaps her unacceptable behaviour would diminish and be replaced by more positive and appropriate responses.

As class teacher I felt quite daunted by this task and I searched the literature for help. I soon realised that Ann had most probably been offering us pre-intentional communication for several months, and that so far the staff had failed to recognise these signals as communication. The pre-intentional communication is 'the information that care-givers, teachers and others can decode from the behaviour of people not yet intentionally sending messages' (Goldbart 1994).

It seemed that Ann had tried and failed to communicate, so that she now tried more extreme behaviours which the staff could not ignore, and which were absolutely certain to elicit a response from someone! This realisation was uncomfortable. I wondered just how many signals I had ignored or failed to notice and with what consequences. This revelation hit me hard and was to be the catalyst for a tremendous change. Not as I had first thought, a change in Ann and her behaviour, but a complete shift of emphasis to a change in me and my behaviour!

As I tried to come to terms with this new insight I chanced upon a book which was to have further repercussions on me and a profound effect upon my whole approach to communication. That book was *Access to Communication* by Nind and Hewett (1994), which gives in great detail an approach they call Intensive Interaction. I was delighted to read: 'If we aim to respond sensitively to each behaviour as an initiation or communicative act we are likely to help our learners to become communicators' (Nind and Hewett 1994: 15). I had already resolved that when I next observed Ann I would be especially vigilant for any signals that could be interpreted as communication.

To present the reader with a clear picture of what happened over the next few months I will summarise Ann's behaviour as it appeared at the beginning of the autumn term in 1995, before any intervention programme was set up with the introduction of Intensive Interaction, and then try to evaluate critically where we had got to and which factors led us to proceed in a new direction.

Summary of Ann's behaviour – September 1995

After an initial period of adjustment to a new classroom, some new staff, and an inevitable change of routine, I observed Ann for a week and noted the following:

'Ann frequently entered school in a tearful and agitated state. Once in the classroom she would continue in her mood and try to cause physical harm to herself (biting her hand), or to others (throwing chairs or equipment), or by trying to destroy her environment (ripping displays from walls and so on).'

It was observed that once Ann was in one of these 'moods', the classroom staff found it quite difficult to calm her down. The negative behaviour could last for up to 30 minutes before Ann could be pacified. Her removal from the classroom was often the only answer. Ann was a child who was quite resistant to eye contact and often would turn away and hide if she accidentally made such contact with a member of staff. She also enjoyed retreating under a blanket or under her own clothes. It appeared, on the surface, that she enjoyed her own isolation. It was noted (during observation) that she spent a great deal of time in her own company banging the window, or on the edge of the group rocking and clapping. These quieter episodes were interspersed with periods of frantic physical activity when Ann would rush around the room attracting attention by loud shouts, claps and behaviour that she knew would get a response from staff.

From the author's observation a pattern seemed to emerge. If left to her own devices Ann appeared unable to find anything constructive to do, but instead would involve herself in one or more of the following behaviours:

- clearing surfaces around the room by throwing apparatus to the floor;
- systematically emptying drawers, cupboards and boxes of books, toys, etc.;
- climbing up onto cupboards or chairs to clear shelves and surfaces;
- banging windows with a flat hand.

Inevitably one or more of these activities resulted in staff intervention. Ann would be led away from the unacceptable activity and encouraged to participate in a more appropriate one. This intervention frequently caused Ann immediate distress and would trigger the cycle of hitting, biting and screaming, as described earlier. Therefore, at first glance, it seemed that Ann's pattern of behaviour was being caused purely by the unwanted intervention of staff, who were interfering with her choice of activity!

With hindsight, however, I now feel that this was not always the case, but that her behaviour was her attempt to communicate, and Ann was beginning to realise which of her behaviours would elicit staff response. However, when she was given attention she did not understand, and had not learned an appropriate response, she reacted in the ways she did. Following the week of observation the class staff met to identify their priorities for the year, and the following were to affect Ann directly:

1. to organise the classroom to provide an inviting, manageable and stimulating environment (this included the removal of Ann's old chair).
2. to organise a structured daily routine within which one member of staff would always be 'available' to Ann to monitor her actions, allowing her independence without disruption or danger to herself or others;
3. to observe and assess Ann's communication skills and monitor the patterns of her behaviour;
4. to address Ann's individual needs by reviewing her individual education programme (IEP);
5. to offer a broad and balanced curriculum which was supported by a 'total communication environment' throughout (Fergusson 1994: 75);
6. to offer a more responsive environment, where any signals from Ann would be seen as communicative and treated as such, and to introduce Intensive Interaction as another 'way in'.

Over the following weeks these six priorities were to prove of great significance in the way things were to develop. Some were even earth shattering!

The intervention programme

The intervention programme was not something that was designed by staff and then imposed upon Ann. It evolved over several weeks as members of staff experimented with ways to encourage and develop the quality of their own interaction and communication with her. The six priorities already identified by class staff were now included in the intervention programme and made up its basic constituents.

Priority 1

To organise the classroom to provide an inviting, manageable and stimulating environment (this included the removal of Ann's old chair)

The classroom was arranged with:

- a group working area;
- a computer area;
- an unstimulating confined workstation (especially designed to keep Ann at her task);
- a book corner, comfortable and secluded;
- an area where Ann could retreat with large soft cushion and blanket;
- a 'ball tent', where Ann could find space and isolation;
- an outside playground, with access from the classroom, used as a reward.

As part of the classroom changes it was decided to remove Ann's old chair. This was a large, cumbersome object with a wooden tray which was not in sympathy with the new classroom style. Staff had used it in previous years to manage a very challenging class, and although it had never been used deliberately to repress Ann, its very presence had a restricting effect on her. Ann had also used the chair herself as a retreat especially after an episode of uncontrollable emotion. I was aware when we made the decision to remove Ann's chair that this would be an important step, as we were changing her environment and interfering with the coping strategies she had set up for herself. However, I had not recognised the significance of the decision, and I was not prepared for the 'domino effect' which was to follow. Without her chair Ann was inevitably compelled to tolerate much more physical contact with staff. I also recognized that I had begun to use myself as a path to defuse some of Ann's difficult emotional outbursts, rather than using the impersonal wooden chair. In other words both Ann and I became more 'accessible' to each other, and there were many more opportunities for us to interact. I found myself much more aware of Ann's attempts to communicate, and thus 'closer contact can facilitate the ability to pick up signals' (Nind and Hewett 1994: 48). Allied to this was a decision to employ more staff to manage the new situation thus fulfilling part of our second priority.

Priority 2

To organise a structured daily routine within which one member of staff would always be 'available' to Ann to monitor her actions, allowing her independence without disruption or danger to herself or others.

After discussion with the school's management team, where I explained the new classroom approach I was allocated three members of staff (including myself) for the morning sessions. This meant that there could always be one person responsible for, and available to, Ann. I decided that the staff would take turns at this, to give Ann access and opportunity to interact with each one of us, and also to give the staff a break from a very demanding task. Having organised the staff, we then devised a daily routine for Ann which was structured to give a balance between periods of 'expectation' when Ann would be encouraged to sit and keep to task, interspersed with periods of relative freedom.

Example of newly structured day

Showing the balance between structured work sessions where expectations were placed on Ann, and sessions of 'free choice'.

Morning session (this was staffed by three adults)

8.50	Enter classroom
	Hang up coat and bag with staff support.
9.00–9.15	Structured activity
	Staff would encourage Ann to choose an activity from the table and sit with her to complete the task. Once completed she was allowed to 'go'.
9.15–9.20	Time for space
	Ann allowed to move freely around room – staff available for intervention if necessary.
9.20–9.40	Hello/good morning session
	Ann encouraged to join the group and sit next to staff for the whole of this session. (During this time Ann was to play the chime bar with the name song, and choose her photo' from the board, select pudding from photos and symbols chart).
9.40–10.00	Time for space
	Ball tent would also be available for use here.
10.00–10.20	Individual objectives (Maths, English)
	One-to-one in specially designed unstimulating work corner. A limit of one or two work tasks to be completed before being allowed to 'go'.
10.20–10.25	Time for space
10.25–10.30	Coat on and out to play
10.30–10.45	Break time in playground
10.45–11.00	Drinks time
	Ann to sit at table with group. To use symbol to indicate drink or biscuit. Choose orange or blackcurrant using bottles. Use an electronic switch to ask for 'more' (only small pieces of a biscuit given at a time).
11.00–11.20	Individual objectives (Maths and English see 10.00–10.20 earlier)
11.20–11.40	Time for space
	Ball tent also available.
11.40–11.58	Quiet time with whole class
	Ann would be expected to be part of this.
11.58	Lunch song and bell
	Ann would be expected to be part of this – using song, apron and bell, as objects of reference to indicate lunch time.
12.00–1.30	Lunch time.
	Cooked meal provided for everyone. Followed by 'playtime' (outdoors, weather permitting).

197

Afternoon session (this was staffed by two adults – and so affected what could be achieved)

1.30–2.15   First structured teaching session (National Curriculum subjects)

Ann was expected to join the group for all sessions where the task had been differentiated to give her access. If this was inappropriate due to her 'mood' then she would work within the classroom on her sensory curriculum with one adult.

2.15–3.00   Second structured teaching session

If Ann had sat for the first session she would now be allowed freedom to choose her own activity for this session – again supported by one adult if necessary.

3.00–3.20   Quiet time/story/singing/preparation for leaving/toileting

'Going home song', and bell (these again being used as objects of reference to anticipate 'home time').

The two decisions (to remove Ann's chair and to allocate a member of staff to be 'available' for Ann every morning) proved to be far more significant than I could ever have imagined at the time. At the outset these decisions were only intuitively felt to be right, and certainly not seen as being of great consequence. However, once implemented, these decisions had an immediate effect upon Ann. Without the barrier of her chair she began to respond to us, and because there were three of us who were more available, interaction was more possible. Also, with an extra team member we could now far more easily implement the decisions.

Priority 3

To observe and assess Ann's communication skills and monitor the patterns of her behaviour.

I observed her for six weeks whenever it was my turn to be 'available' for her, to determine 'where Ann was'. I watched her closely on other occasions, such as during playtime, dinner time, and during group sessions when I was not taking the lead. It was soon apparent that Ann was already using some communication that could be classified as 'non-verbal strategy' (Goldbart 1994: 15).

This included:

- eye contact, (very rarely);
- physical contact, usually initiated by the staff and tolerated by Ann;
- attention-seeking behaviour (sometimes), usually in the form of inappropriate behaviour, such as removing her clothes;
- indicating a preference at drinks time by picking up a cup or a biscuit placed in front of her;
- requesting, by climbing up onto a chair to reach the biscuit tin (on two separate occasions).

This discovery made me realise that although I had known Ann for about nine months my knowledge of her was quite 'patchy'. I had to admit to myself that up to now I really had not made a relationship with her of any quality or meaning. I really did not know this child, for up to now there had been a barrier between us. However, this situation was about to change because in observing and being available to her destined a dramatic effect on the situation! Having read Nind and Hewett's (1994) book *Access to Communication* I approached these periods of observation with specific attitudes in mind. I attempted to adopt some of the basic features that are central to an Intensive Interactive approach. These included sensitivity, responsiveness, attentiveness, imitation and physical contact. Although my chief intention at this time had been to be an observer, I soon began to realise that this was asking the impossible of both myself and Ann, as these extracts from my observation diary well illustrate:

Day 1   Ann was sitting on the carpet playing with a ring stacker. I positioned myself nearby, down on the floor at her level, but far enough away to be non-threatening. Ann began several sideways glances in my direction showing an awareness of my presence. I reciprocated but each time we made eye contact, Ann immediately looked away. After five minutes Ann got up and walked away.

Day 6   The same situation as last week, but Ann was playing with a pillow case and a mitten. After the usual few seconds of eye contact which had developed over the past week, today it was accompanied by a pink tongue being popped out at me. I imitated. Ann copied and a game ensured. This lasted about one minute and Ann ended it in her usual manner by walking away.

Day 7   Same eye contact as yesterday, I initiated the tongue popping game, Ann imitated! I followed. Duration, three minutes.

Day 10 Ann really wanted closer physical contact. She approached me and seemed ready to start the 'tongue game' (although she waited for me to lead). Other dramatic occurrences today:

  – she came closer,
  – she sat down beside me,
  – I place my hand on her knee. She imitated.
  – she placed her hand on my knee,
  – she moved her chair to a better position.
  – Quality interaction had occurred.
  – Over the next few weeks other observations of Ann included:

  • she was calmer for more of the time,
  • she was more tolerant of adult intervention;
  • she was beginning to make and maintain eye contact in one-to-one situations;
  • staff were able to pacify her more quickly;
  • Ann was showing signs of 'enjoying' physical contact.

Priority 4

To address Ann's individual needs by reviewing her IEP.

Staff hoped that by developing Ann's communication skills her disruptive behaviour would decrease. Thus communication became the priority in the short term, and Ann's IEP was reviewed with this in mind. Enjoyable activities promoting communication skills were increased and situations and circumstances that could lead to the undesirable behaviours were reduced. A list of objectives for mathematics and English would be worked on daily (in the quiet workstation area) and broken down into easily achievable goals. These would always take place after negotiation with Ann, and the instruction, 'Do this piece and then you can go'. Ann's reward would be 'time for space' once all her tasks were completed. All the activities promoted 'looking and listening' skills, including matching and sorting, in order to develop her visual discrimination and so help with her symbol recognition. Other forms of stimulation included:

- music (which provided a mean of non-verbal communication);
- sensory experiences (to encourage tolerance of physical contact and to develop interaction);
- massage (Aromatherapy 'Tac Pac' [a 'Tac Pac' is a 'sensory package which can be used in a one-to-one situation; it includes music, massage, and many tactile experiences.]);
- sessions in the sensory room were also timetabled and seen as being beneficial to Ann;
- access to the National Curriculum, using differentiation – this often included sensory activities of all kinds.

It was decided that Intensive Interaction would also be included to develop Ann's communication skills. Staff felt that at first it should be used spontaneously and intuitively in any situation that occurred rather than timetabled as a formal programme, and so a period of interactive play ensued and was included into daily routines.

The introduction of Intensive Interaction was to prove another catalyst with far reaching consequences. Eighteen months after its introduction, when Ann was 7 years old, a formal programme of Intensive Interaction was undertaken with a new interactive partner which has proved very worthwhile, and after two years and with a new staff team (at the time of writing), it continues to show a beneficial effect.

Priority 5

To offer a broad and balanced curriculum which was supported by a 'total communication environment' throughout (Fergusson 1994)

Staff attempted to set up within the classroom situation an environment which fulfilled the criteria recommended by Fergusson for example:

Criterion 1: 'offer frequent and consistent opportunities to communicate'. We expected Ann to join in several communication sessions during the day, for example, when saying 'Hello', or when indicating at drinks time her choices and preferences, when choosing a pudding from her symbols, and choosing activities from two photographs offered her.

Criterion 2: 'create a need or desire to communicate'. We would present Ann with situations to encourage both her problem-solving skills and motivate her to ask for help (putting her favourite biscuit inside a screw topped container, or giving her an unopened packet of crisps were wonderful ways to achieve this!)

Criterion 3: 'provide access to a means of expression' and 'view all modes/means of communication as having equal value'. We supported speech with every media we could think of, including objects of reference, pictures, photographs, signing 'BIG MACK' ['BIG MACK' is a communication aid used with pre-verbal pupils. It is a large, brightly coloured, touch-sensitive switch which controls a pre-recorded message, e.g. more please, good morning, etc.] and so on.

Criterion 4: 'be consistently responsive to every communicate attempt'. This criterion we found the most difficult to fulfil. In a busy classroom it is very easy to miss certain communicative attempts especially if they are as subtle as a facial expression, an eye movement or a gesture. Then having perceived this as communication, to find the necessary spare attention to respond in a positive way is almost an impossibility. However, we decided to make this our priority, and that we would be sensitive to any signals from Ann and respond to them immediately, clearly and consistently. With hindsight this was a very significant step, for although we found it very demanding, it soon became apparent that a two-way process was occurring and we were becoming the 'reinforcers'. I recorded all these reinforcers to discover which ones could be incorporated into the intervention programme, and used to reward appropriate responses and behaviours!

Ann's reinforcers

Category 1 – objects:

- biscuits;
- drinks;
- crisps (especially the packets);
- 'scrunchies' (elasticated hairbands);
- small objects (to be carried about);
- sensory bag (pillow case full of tactile materials – bubble wrap, sandpaper, foil, etc);

- mittens and gloves.

Category 2 – activities:

- spa pool;
- 'freedom' (in classroom, playground and P.E. hall);
- computer with touch-screen.

Category 3 – attention:

- physical contact;
- cuddles;
- games (chases, rough-and-tumble);
- praise;
- staff.

Priority 6

To offer a more responsive environment, where any signals from Ann would be seen as communicative, and treated as such, and to introduce Intensive Interaction as another 'way in'.

I have already explained in Priority 5 how we tried to create a more responsive environment for Ann, and how this began to affect her responsiveness. However, in all our dealings with Ann and with all the different techniques we attempted, the most significant was the introduction of Intensive Interaction, for the effects it had on Ann (and us!), and her acquisition of communication skills.

Moving on

January 1996

We decided from the outset that we would introduce 'interactive play' within Ann's normal daily routine. Initially this would be initiated by one of us in a formal work situation and then spontaneity would be allowed to take over. I have previously described how this had already begun to take place incidentally during my periods of observation, well before any formal intervention programme had been introduced. So the seeds of Intensive Interaction had been already sown before the programme was up and running. When we began the intervention programme Ann was not initiating any physical contact with me, but she was making eye contact and tolerating my closeness to her.

March 1996

I decided to try and elicit a response from Ann by using her favourite toys. The following notes from an interactive play session show how this was eventually achieved. The classroom was empty, except for Ann and myself. I encouraged Ann to join me on the carpet in the corner of the room with her favourite 'noisy' pillow case. Within this were her preferred items, e.g. a wailing tube (a piece of plastic which when swung around made a howling noise), some Indian bells attached to a strap, a sorting box with shapes that whine when replaced correctly, a bath-book with a squeaker, and a yogurt pot full of lentils. Ann showed no interest in joining me but lay on the carpet a little way off, casting a glance to see what I was doing. I began to unload the bag one item at a time, expressing loudly to anyone who would listen (hopefully Ann) what wonderful discoveries I was making. I then proceeded to play with each item. After a few minutes I was aware that I had Ann's full attention and that she had moved much closer to me to gain a better view. I continued playing with the wailing tube but this time I blew through it directing my breath at her. She responded by giggling so I did it again, but moved much closer to her. A game ensued, gathering momentum as it went. The whole episode lasted only two or three minutes, but I felt that we had started to communicate. The 'mutual enjoyment' between Ann and myself had been the breakthrough. This echoed the discovery by Nind and Hewett (1994: 6) 'Pleasure first and foremost'.

Referring again to Nind and Hewett's book, I was reminded about 'picking up and following cues' (Nind and Hewett 1994: 52). I had begun doing this instinctively, but found its significance from my reading.

May 1996

Within weeks of the first really playful encounter with the wailing tube, Ann initiated her first of many interactive games, which was achieved by my 'picking up' and 'following' her cues. Here is a brief account of what occurred:

- Ann approached me and indicated by making eye contact that she wanted my attention.
- I responded with eye contact.
- I placed my face close to her (this necessitated my kneeling down).
- Ann raised her arms.
- I copied.
- She brought her arms down onto my shoulders.
- I imitated and placed my arms around her middle.
- Still we held eye contact.
- Suddenly with no warning Ann left eye contact and hugged me close.
- In the same split second Ann slipped her hand slyly around my neck.
- She suddenly grabbed the '*scrunchie' from my hair (* a headband).
- Ann ran away, laughing.
- I followed.
- A chase ensued, with anticipation and laughter.

- Ann dropped the scrunchie.
- I followed, picked it up and returned it to my head.
- I resumed my seat at the table.
- Ann circled the room, watching me closely.
- Within a minute Ann wandered past me and whisked the scrunchie away again.
- The game was repeated.

This was the very first time Ann had initiated a game.

As the weeks progressed 'the scrunchie game' became Ann's way of indicating her readiness for interaction. The objects have changed (mittens in a coat pocket is now her favourite), and the action can be more prolonged or take a different direction, but her readiness to interact is always signalled in a similar way.

Over the past 18 months these games have become a prominent feature of her repertoire. In fact this is very much a daily ritual on the playground and no one is quite sure who her next 'victim' will be. In recent weeks Ann has extended this interaction to include her peers who respond with equal delight to their 'new-found friend'.

As Ann's willingness to interact began to increase staff were in bouyant mood about the positive changes that were occurring. However, I do not want to give the impression that all of Ann's previously challenging behaviour had been totally replaced by this new positive response. Her co-operative, playful episodes were certainly increasing, but were interspersed with longer periods of uncontrollable anger and distress which still had to be managed. Helping Ann through these difficult times was a demanding task, and only possible because staff took turns throughout the day to be available for Ann; sometimes in the role of a playful interactive partner and at other times as a steady calming influence during the more turbulent times.

Personally I found this a very frustrating and emotionally draining experience. Ann's mood swings were very dramatic and appeared to have no particular trigger. Having shared with her the joy of close human contact, her periods of isolation and distress seemed all the worse. There followed a period of several weeks when Ann's health deteriorated and her epilepsy took control. I felt that this possibly could account for her recent dramatic mood swings and decided that once she was well again I needed to take some positive steps to regain control of what had become a difficult situation. In the meantime the staff tried to maintain an equilibrium to support her through her illness. Once Ann was well again I took several steps to better manage her more difficult days. I introduced a daily observation chart where staff could record each and every incident – the time, the trigger, the situation and consequences of every mood swing, to try to discover whether there was any pattern to Ann's behaviour. It was apparent that as consistent an approach as possible would be a sensible way forward, and so with staff agreement I put into place some basic management strategies to handle Ann's outbursts. The choice of which technique to use at any time would be based upon the severity of the outbursts and danger to herself or others. These included the following.

In order to establish communication:

- approach Ann calmly with a steady, soothing voice, and remove any physical dangers or provocations;
- maintain eye contact with Ann;
- offer close physical contact;
- cuddle her;
- maintain close physical proximity, i.e. go and 'be with' Ann both emotionally and physically;
- massage her back, hold hands, etc.;
- try a distraction technique to return Ann to more appropriate activities;
- in extreme situations when she was in danger of hurting herself, 'enfold' her firmly until she is calm (I prefer to use the term 'enfold' rather than 'hold' as it implies protection rather than restraint);
- maintain communication at all times;
- try to have an empathetic awareness of her feelings;
- stay calm and do not allow your own behaviour or feelings to interfere in the process;
- once the episode has subsided, take Ann for a quiet calm walk away from the classroom, continually reassuring, in readiness to return to the classroom situation once more.

In order to establish a consistency to this routine, I decided that at the end of each day staff would try to find time to discuss the day's occurrences. This helped to iron out any problems that arose and also gave all of us opportunities to express our fears and anxieties. This proved a useful way to gain mutual support, and I recommend such a method to those wishing to venture on similar programmes. However, in the dynamics of a busy classroom it is not always possible for staff to meet together at the end of the day.

Another vital factor in the management of the situation was the keeping of well-documented records, especially of our observations. Staff discovered that when we analysed the records we found that there were three times during the day when Ann was at her most difficult. These were first thing in the morning, the session following lunch time, and just before home time. An awareness of this led us to make certain decisions about levels of staffing to try to avoid confrontations with Ann. The result of this is that we gave her 'one to one' quality time, timetabled for the times of the day we expected her to be most difficult, to try to diffuse any conflicts before they arose. Of course, we did not always get this right – either because Ann changed her pattern, or because staff had other unscheduled demands upon their time.

By January 1997 it was quite obvious that Intensive Interaction had provided Ann with a new way of communicating. She was generally calmer in herself and much more willing to participate in group activities, as well as tolerating activities in a one-to-one situation for longer periods. Challenging behaviour and disruptive outbursts still occurred but with the newly established relationship with staff these were becoming far less frequent and were more easily diffused.

With a change of class staff it was decided to set up a more structured Intensive Interaction programme for Ann. From January to March 1997 the sessions continued to be spontaneous and happened only when Ann indicated she wanted them. However, as the months progressed Ann began to show a definite preference towards one interactive partner. She also demonstrated that she was benefiting positively from this new relationship, I therefore decided to develop the session into a much more structured activity. From April 1997 there was a daily timetabled session of Intensive Interaction outside the classroom with her chosen interactive partner. This took place as soon as she arrived at school (one of the times of day she found most difficult). Although this placed extra pressures on the rest of the staff (the class was now without one of the assistants) the benefits began to outweigh the costs. It was soon obvious that on those days when we were unable to give the timetabled Intensive Interaction session that Ann was less able to manage her own behaviour for the rest of the day and that her outbursts would escalate.

Progress and problems

By June 1997 Ann was showing great progress in her interaction abilities, and had gained new communication skills such as imitation, initiation, anticipation and turn-taking. She was also sitting with the class at particular times of the day, and at least during some part of every lesson. She was frequently requesting objects (drinks, activities, etc.) by dragging a member of staff to the appropriate cupboard or shelf and demanding her preferred items. She was also requesting time out of the classroom by taking a member of staff's hand and dragging them to the door and to the P.E. hall or playground. However, at the same time (and this should not be surprising) her tolerance levels seemed to diminish resulting in more frequent temper tantrums and a new repertoire of disruptive behaviour.

A new behaviour management programme had to be tried to see if Ann's disruptions could be replaced with something more appropriate. At this time (June 1997) Ann was beginning to enjoy being with her friends and was definitely a part of the class, freely choosing to sit with fellow class members several times each day. In trying to find a way through Ann's latest disruptive behaviour, one member of the staff suggested that perhaps we should remove Ann's new found enjoyment of being part of the class, as a way of helping her manage her own behaviour. After much discussion the following behavioural management programme was put in place.

Ann's Behaviour Management Programme June 1997

Disruptive behaviour
This term covers the following behaviours:

- running around the classroom;

- sweeping items from surfaces;
- attempting to empty cupboards;
- throwing items.

Coping strategy to be followed:

1. Staff will approach Ann and say 'No Ann, or you go outside' in a firm loud voice. Then present Ann with a choice of two activities she likes in an attempt to distract her.
2. If Ann continues in her disruptive behaviour, staff say 'Go outside, Ann', and take her outside the patio door and leave her for 30 seconds only. Then Ann is brought back into the classroom, praising her and offering her physical closeness.
3. Continue with number 1 as necessary.

The above strategy will also be applied if Ann is behaving in a way that may affect the safety of herself and others. All incidents of Ann being removed from the classroom will be recorded on an antecedent, behaviour, consequences (ABC) chart. Regular discussions between class staff will take place and Ann's parents will receive copies of the recording sheet. Their comments will be welcomed.

Alternative activities

It is essential that while we are saying 'No' to Ann, a range of alternative activities are made available to her. Such activities may involve the 'feelie' and 'noisy' pillow cases, which are favourites and several 'play boxes' with specific items which motivate Ann.

Ann's behaviour programme was in use for the last four weeks of the summer term. At first our guess that she did not like being away from us (albeit for only 30 seconds at a time) seemed to be correct. After only a short time Ann seemed to realise what was expected of her, and that certain of her actions had its consequences.

After the first few days it seemed that just one warning was sufficient to persuade Ann to change her behaviour. However several days later she seemed to have forgotten all that she learnt, and her behaviour became unpredictable once more; and she was again persistent in her attempts to disrupt the classroom. We began to wonder whether she was enjoying her 30 seconds outside, although her body language seemed to indicate the contrary. During the following week she allowed staff to distract her by the more motivating activities, and thus seemed to be avoiding the 30 second exclusion. But the next week she again proved far less predictable; this was the last few days of the summer term. In trying to make some sense of Ann's behaviour, one or two considerations need attention:

- a month's trial gave insufficient data to draw any firm conclusions;
- there were too many variable factors, for example, the quality of the distracting activities, and the consistency of approach because of the number of staff involved;
- there is a suspicion that the changes observed in Ann were less to do with

Ann's ability to communicate and more to do with staff's imposing their will on her!

Looking back over the two and a half years I have worked with Ann, there has been tremendous change in both Ann and also in myself. For Ann it has been a period when she has begun to develop new communication skills. She has perceived that by using these effectively she is able to control her environment, her learning and the people around her. She has discovered a new enjoyment of life and has become more socially involved. Anne has acquired some of the true basics of communication. She is now able to imitate, anticipate, initiate interactive games and thoroughly enjoy physical closeness. She is a much more open, warm and affectionate human being, responsive to a wide variety of people and situations. She is calmer, more controlled and generally more tolerant of those around her. She is able to sit willingly with the class group for longer, participating at a level relevant to her and showing an obvious delight in her new-found friends.

For me it has been a time of enlightenment: my presuppositions have been challenged and some attitudes fundamentally shifted. I have also had to learn and develop sensitivities, heightened perception and awareness. I have also had to live with the feelings of frustration and failure and accept that some of Ann's learning difficulties lay not only with her but also with me. I have learnt to accept that it was my inability to 'tune in' to her 'where she was' that was an important part of the barrier. Through all this I have come to a profound realisation that as well as being an educator I have become the central tool or instrument within this interactive partnership by which interaction has taken place.

Working with Ann has been a quite remarkable experience. I have been privileged to share warmth and solidarity with a fellow human being at her speed and very much on her terms. This partnership has been based on acceptance and openness, value and respect. To have shared such a relationship with a child is a precious privilege. Ann has now moved on to a new class and I hope taken with her a little of the joy we discovered together. I know that I will take with me many things I have learnt from Ann.

References

Fergusson, A. (1994) 'Planning for communication', in Rose, R., Fergusson, A., Coles, C., Byers, R., Banes, D. (eds) *Implementing the Whole Curriculum for Pupils with Learning Difficulties*. London: David Fulton Publishers.

Goldbart, J. (1994) 'Opening the communication curriculum to students with PMLD's', in Ware, J. (ed) *Educating Children with Profound and Multiple Learning Difficulties*. London: David Fulton Publishers.

Nind, M. and Hewett, D. (1994) *Access to Communication: Developing the Basics of Communication with People with Severe Learning Difficulties Through Intensive Interaction*. London: David Fulton Publishers.

Chapter 12

Exotic communication, conversations and scripts – or tales of the pained, the unheard and the unloved

Geraint Ephraim

Introduction

I suspect that the relationship between carers of people with a learning disability and clinical psychologists has often been a sort of love – hate thing. An old hospital institution joke used to be: 'If you want to kill a few hours ask a clinical psychologist what his (always his, never her) role is'. Yet there has always been a hope that one day the carer might come across a clinical psychologist with all the answers. All this is at the level of myth. No one has all the answers. Most people's reality is that individual clinical psychologists have helped to some degree, or have been useless.

A hitch-hiker's guide to clinical psychology might start, 'There are two types of clinical psychologists . . . Listeners . . . and . . . Doers'. In the 1960s clinical psychologists used to be the handmaidens of psychiatrists and would dutifully provide intelligence quotient (IQ) figures to confirm the psychiatrist's estimation (which was usually pretty good). Then psychologists remembered their initial training when they did their first degree and introduced learning theory in the shape of behaviour modification. Their God was B. F. Skinner. They proved that people with a learning disability could learn – clinical psychologists became doers. They brought realistic and optimistic technologies into the field. They acquired power through this and yet, being essentially pragmatic, they took onboard the idea that nursing staff were quite capable of using this technology. They then took a thundering leap and became nursing staff trainers. Despite this wonderful altruism they maintained a position of superiority by retaining clinical ownership of the more complex cases.

I came into clinical psychology and learning disability (mental subnormality in those days) from a background in child care. I'd done stuff like child development, sensitivity groups, therapeutic communities and contemplated personal analysis. I'd even shaken hands with Donald Winnicott, one of the founding fathers of British psychoanalytic childcare theory. So understandably, I hated the controlling nature of behaviourism. Yet, 20 years on, some of my closest colleagues are radical behaviourists. I don't understand them, they use a different language from myself, yet I never cease to be surprised about how much we agree in practice.

The language I use is based on a framework that helps me to have some sort of direction when I am expected to be of help. A lot of this framework comes from my experience in child care. I have some understanding of how the infant with a disability can affect his carers. I also have ideas about how the disabled infant will follow his or her own manner of development which is similar but not identical to that of a normal infant. My understanding of normal development comes from academic heroes like Piaget, Bruner and Vygotsky. I have psychoanalytic heroes like Winnicott and Bowlby. In my style of working Carl Rogers is an important influence (Rogers 1990).

I have always found it useful to engage directly with the client. I've experienced anger in trying to feed a controlling and manipulative child with cerebral palsy. She spat food out of her mouth and, despite being athetoid, she could accurately hit the plate off the table to the floor. This provided insight and respect into staff feelings. I remember walking hand-in-hand with a child with autism, imitating his gait and giving him control over where he went. I remember tuning into the quiet fun he had listening to the sounds of his own feet walking through autumn leaves.

I suspect that Dave Hewett invited me to write a chapter because I can produce snappy titles which he likes. The title is 14 words long but it is a very brief synopsis of the next several thousand words. The words 'the pained, the unheard and the unloved' represent as simple a framework as possible to help understand the very broad, rich, yet tragic range of human experience which is labelled challenging behaviour. The words 'exotic communication, conversations and scripts' provide a second simple framework, superimposed upon the first which looks at how we relate to one another. The word 'tale' promises a story, hopefully entertaining, hopefully enlightening, which plays out some of the very rich and complex interaction between the two frameworks. The tale is also partially autobiographical but also reflects my current interests and preoccupation. I too have my scripts which I have already declared in this introduction.

Theories and perceptions

Many years ago when I was still a baby psychologist, I had the honour to meet a young man named Edward. He was about 18 years old, had severe learning disabilities and had no speech. He was strikingly handsome, fit, agile and big. He was very big. There were times when he became quite disturbed and could be violent. Staff working on the ward where he lived were very wary, even frightened of him, and during his psychotic outbursts it was reputed that it took six male members of staff to hold him down!

Edward attended the hospital school. He was in a class of about eight youngsters and the classroom was staffed by a teacher and classroom assistant, both female. They recognised that when he was under any sort of pressure he would begin to puff air through his pursed lips. They realised that he seemed under pressure when he didn't understand what was going on or what was expected of him. They took pains to help him with this. If they failed to do this he would have an outburst. Occasionally one of the two members of staff was hit. Despite this they were not frightened of him. They had a theory that allowed them to explain and often predict his behaviour. The ward staff's psychotic formulation defined him as unpredictable and irrational. It was the unpredictability that made the ward staff nervous.

Years later, Graham Fawcett (another psychologist friend) drew my attention to the work of two linguists, Sperber and Wilson (1986). They turned linguistics on its head. Until then theories of communication had placed the onus for successful communication on the person transmitting the message. We have an image of a mouth with tons and tons of information coming out of it. This information pours into a passive ear which is like a bucket holding all these tons of information. In Sperber and Wilson's view, things are different. We radiate information all the time. We do this through words, gestures, body posture, movement, etc. Their term for this is 'ostending', as in ostentatious. Communication happens when the listener attends to and interprets our ostentions. I might say 'I agree with you'. If however, my fists are clenched and there is a tightness in my voice, my listener might understand that I am not agreeing with him. If I say 'It's a bit drafty where I'm sitting' he might understand me to say 'Shut the window!'. The interpretation is based on the listener's knowledge of the other person, their situation etc. Sperber and Wilson termed this 'encyclopaedic knowledge'. It is the listener that bears the onus for successful communication. In Edward's story, the classroom staff enabled understanding through their reading of his behaviour and this reading was informed by their theories about him.

As I slowly grew up to become a clinical psychologist, I had numerous experiences along the lines suggested by Edward's story. I often worked in situations where staff were demoralised, unsupported, and coping with very difficult clients. I also realised that what I had to offer seemed very limited given the limited resources that staff often worked with. It's cliché, but I had no magic wands. What I tended to offer was an attempt to understand the client. This seemed most useful when this attempt was shared with staff. What I brought into the situation was based on theories of infant and child development. Staff brought in their knowledge and experience of the client and their relationship with that client. When a client engaged in challenging behaviour, staff perception of the severity of the problem was linked to their understanding of the reasons behind the behaviour.

Behaviour as communication

The term challenging behaviour was initially coined to help staff to think of difficult behaviour, not so much as a problem but as a challenge to services. Unfortunately the term has now acquired pejorative meaning. New labels are often invented to replace pejorative ones. So let me suggest that there is no such thing as challenging behaviour. What we have is exotic communication. (No doubt if this term caught on it would itself become pejorative and someone else will come along with another bright linguistic idea like 'offensive ostentations'.) A punch in the face is an act of communication which is very difficult not to hear. Its effect may be heard but the message behind the punch may not have been listened to, let alone be understood.

From communication to conversations

So far I have used the word communication as if it were a parcel that one person virtually throws at the other. If they're not attending, the parcel will hit the receiver in the head and it will hurt. It hurts 'cos they ain't been listening. If they're attending then they will catch the parcel and they won't be hurt. Communication described in this way implies power. The person chucking the parcel has a lot of power. In the culture of care work, empowering is a good thing but the power that the exotic communicator has does not mean that they are happy. In a sense that sort of power can add to a person's unhappiness. The recipient of the parcel is essentially passive. If the parcel hits us, we can be frightened. We can become angry. In our anger we might start throwing parcels back. We have become exotic communicators!

Let's contrast communication as an expression of power with a special form of communication which we call a conversation. In a conversation, both participants are equals. There is no power struggle, no domination – the participants share. They value each other and they value the conversation for its own sake, simply because it is fun. Approaches such as Intensive Interactions (Nind and Hewett 1994, see also Ephraim 1986, Caldwell and Flynn 1995, Caldwell 1996) provide a framework for valuing and promoting conversations, especially with people who have little or no language and limited social interest.

I implied earlier that the theories that carers have about their clients predetermine their perception of their clients and the client's communications. A wrong theory, such as the theory that Edward was psychotic, prevents understanding and conversation. The absence of a theory can be equally non-facilitating. We need theories or frameworks that help us arrive at a useful understanding of the individual. It is this understanding that allows us to interpret the others' ostentations and make conversations possible. But people are complex and changing and no one theory will do the job. So if our aim is to understand then we must be open to exploring the usefulness of different frameworks. The richer our understanding then the richer will be our conversations.

Venn and the exotic 'Why?'

Some years ago I had a series of conversations with a nursing colleague, Paul Baker, about some of the many clients that we had been working with and the idea of why people 'challenge'. Suddenly some bubbles formed in my head, joined together and got labelled. This is a condition that several psychologists over the years have suffered and is called vennphilia. This is an obsession with drawing overlapping circles. Each circle represents a category and things that belong to more than one category are represented in the overlap of circles. These overlapping circles are called Venn diagrams. The sort of psychologist that is prone to vennphilia tends to be rather fuzzier and cuddlier than those psychologists who are more hard-nosed, rational and posessing a well-developed procedural framework. Fuzzy psychologists sometimes feel guilty about their lack of certainty, so something like a Venn diagram serves as a pretension that they are in control and understand what they talk about. Along with vennphilia comes the delusion that everything can be explained by pictures of intersecting circles. My particular delusion can be seen in Figure 12.1.

The three circles represent the idea that people who communicate exotically may be in pain, or may not be listened to, or may have longstanding difficulties with love and relationships. The intersections of the circles represent the idea that in individual cases any of these three things may interact.

Those in pain

To explain the three circles I'll start by considering those in pain but I'll differentiate between physical and emotional pain. I could represent this by two overlapping circles but that would be over-indulging my vennphilia.

Physical pain

It is very easy to overlook pain as a topic of exotic communication. We can get involved in all manners of theories that overlook simple and often remediable

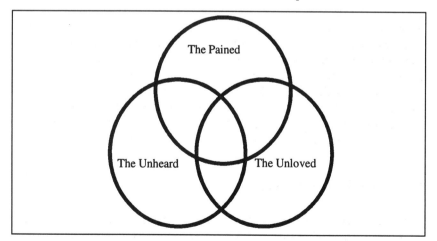

Figure 12.1 My Venn Delusion

sources of pain or discomfort. I'll not attempt a comprehensive list but consider the following: toothache, backache, constipation, uncomfortable shoes. I have experienced all of these. Being a warm and placid person these conditions in themselves did not cause me to engage in exotic communications. However, additional difficulties may cause me to become more irritable, even to become just a little bit snappy. I have the luxury of being able to tell people around me that I'm in pain and they usually modify their interaction to make life less fraught. (In reality they probably avoid me!) I also have the option of going to the doctor to communicate my symptoms and seek actions that will remedy the pain. If I did not have these options then my experience of pain would also be pretty chronic and lonely. It would be very likely that I would become an exotic communicator.

Such causes of pain are relatively commonplace but there are other causes of physical pain which can be less prosaic. People of Afro-Caribbean descent may suffer from sickle cell anaemia. This condition can cause considerable discomfort in the joints. A person suffering from cerebral palsy is likely to have periods of discomfort or pain. If someone is diagnosed as having a particular syndrome it's worthwhile doing some homework and gaining information. A few years ago a young person was referred for his behaviour. It was mentioned that he had 'nail-patella' syndrome. I knew nothing of this condition so I dutifully cadged a text book from a nursing colleague. It turned out that 'nail-patella' syndrome is a genetic condition where finger nails are absent and the knee cap is either very small or absent. The absence of kneecaps had put great stress on his ankles with the obvious result that there were times when he experienced pain or discomfort. In considering physical pain it is as well to obtain the advice of a medic, or a community nurse. Physiotherapists can be very good at pain!

I am a person who respects my body. I like to sit in an armchair with a glass of wine. I do not engage in bizarre activities such as jogging. The people that I know who jog are addicted to it. If they miss one of their sessions, they become irritable, even a bit depressed. Joggers are in fact junkies. When they miss their jog, they miss their fix. They are addicted to their own home-grown potion. The human body, as part of its system to manage pain, has the capacity to create endorphin. This is a drug related to heroin. Jogging is quite a good way to get an endorphin fix. The next time you see a jogger, remember that they are scoring!

If you have a toothache, you may feel that what you want to do is to hit the site of the pain with your fist. What you are instinctively thinking about is how to increase your endorphin levels so as to lessen the experience of pain. It seems very likely that some people who engage in self-injurious behaviour suffer from endorphin addiction. The root of this behaviour may have been a history of toothaches, or earaches. If there is a history of catarrh, sinus problems etc. then this possibility seems very likely. Such self-injurious behaviour is very difficult to manage and causes staff great distress. Advice to ignore such addictive behaviour is ineffective. The effect is that the behaviour continues and staff stress levels are likely to increase. Where the behaviour has this addictive quality then a cold turkey approach advocated in *Gentle Teaching* (McGee *et al.* 1987) seems appropriate. Here, staff block the behaviour by using a cushion or similar to prevent the person inflicting blows upon themselves. There may be a recreational element to such addiction inasmuch as the client is also bored, understimulated etc. For such an approach to be effective, the blocking needs to be extremely vigilant. At the same time the person needs to be engaged in alternative activities that relate to their interests and abilities. Conversations along the lines suggested by interactional approaches are likely to succeed. However, if conversations happen only in response to self-injury, then it seems reasonable to ask for a conversation by hitting yourself. Such behaviour is quite rational and pragmatic especially if pain can give you a buzz. Some practitioners have become interested in blocking the endorphin cycle by the use of drugs such as Naxalone which are normally used for heroine addiction. From the perspective offered here, if there is a basis for such an approach, it would be more effective if the person were given the opportunity for conversations and activities as and when they were in the mood.

This latter statement may cause alarm for carers. They might think, 'Most psychologists tell us to ignore behaviour, this nutter is telling us to provide attention on demand! Forget it!' My own experience of my relationships with other people rarely involves the idea of having to work hard to get their attention. Sometimes, however, I may actively seek someone's attention, maybe across a crowded room with a friend who is so distracted by a multitude of distractions that he is not aware of my presence. If my friend is engrossed in a clearly intimate conversation then I would judge it inappropriate to crash in on his privacy. I would choose my time, confident that I will succeed. The other times I actively attempt to gain someone's attention are when there is some urgent matter that needs attention. Most of the time I take the attention of others completely for granted.

However, here have been times in my life when, for whatever reason, I have felt insecure. During such periods and at their most acute, I may have felt I needed friends' attention. Then I did not take it for granted and was grateful, perhaps surprised, when they listened and even understood. I am able to take attention for granted because it is part of the normal human condition. Most people with learning disabilities have never had the opportunity to develop such security. Many still crave attention because of their insecurities. To use a label such as 'attention-seeking behaviour' and to judge such behaviour 'undesirable' is to deny the person's place as a member of society.

To give such a strong message to carers might make them feel incompetent and guilty. The reality is that, however desirable, giving such unconditional attention is impractical. If the potatoes have boiled and need draining, or the staff rota needs to be completed by 2 p.m., a demand for unconditional attention is very inconvenient. Immediate response to such a demand is impractical.

If a person demands our attention when the potatoes need draining, it seems reasonable for them to wait. It is also reasonable to help them to wait by saying 'let me drain the potatoes then I'll talk to you'. We can actually engage in token conversation whilst draining the potatoes. What is important is that having attended to our own necessities we then turn to the person and engage in conversation. If there is sufficient consistency in this then the other person will know that 'wait' isn't forever, that quite soon they will be engaged in conversation. Where there is certainty that the conversation will happen, waiting is no problem. The attention can be taken for granted. Exotic communication is the communication of the desperate. Convivial conversation is the pastime of the relaxed and confident.

(Under the heading of physical pain include epilepsy on the pretext that pain is a signal of some organic event or process that is damaging or dysfunctional, but I'll discuss epilepsy later.)

Emotional pain

Our lives are full of other people. We are social beings and our world is full of relationships. If a friend or colleague leaves us, we miss them. We can no longer take them for granted. In a sense we might grieve the loss. If someone close to us dies then most certainly we will grieve. Someone's behaviour may well be grief for a member of staff that has moved to another job. They may not understand why or where, but they are missing one of their kith. Addressing this grief may be painful for the carers and understandably they may well deny that the person is missing someone. Such losses and grief become even more painful for carers to share when it is caused by a death. Mary Oswin has written eloquently about these losses (Oswin 1981, 1984) and is well worth reading.

People with a learning disability typically spend significant time together. They share relationships with each other. Often they are treated as a group. The death or departure of a friend or even a member of the group who is not a friend will be painful but it can be mysterious and perplexing to a person who has little or no language.

I remember members of the special needs unit of an ATC who appeared to be struggling to make sense of the absence of a member. This man became increasingly disturbed to the extent that he was admitted to the Learning Disability Hospital that served that area. A matter of months after his admission he died. It would seem perhaps that his medical condition had some connection with his behaviour. After this sad event it seemed that if any member of the special needs group became disturbed in any way then the behaviour of the whole group seemed affected. I had an intuition that the group, though non-verbal, had a theory which seemed to confuse illness and behavioural problems. It felt as if when someone else in the group became disturbed an individual would be frightened of catching it and so be sent away to hospital to die. Such an intuition may be pure fantasy. It may be that just feelings were being transmitted amongst the group without being manifest as coherent thoughts.

For many years the dominant psychology of learning disabilities was behavioural. Behavioural approaches were, and remain, very useful. Yet, when this was the only legitimate viewpoint, it seemed as if people with learning disabilities were only allowed to have behaviour. More recently, following developments in psychological practice in adult mental health, there is developing a cognitive–behavioural approach in working with people with learning disabilities (see Kroese *et al.* 1997). It seems that now people with learning disabilities are beginning to be allowed to have thoughts. Though many practitioners struggle with counselling or psychotherapeutic approaches, there is very little written about it (however, see Sinason 1992). There is a great need for work which addresses the emotional needs of people with a learning disability.

If they are allowed thoughts and feelings then fine, we can talk to them about it if they are articulate and have speech. But what if they understand less than we think they do? Or what if they have no speech. What then? Let's look at the second circle in the Venn diagram

The unheard

I'd like to introduce the reader to Dylan, a most remarkable person. He is in his late 20s and has quite severe learning disabilities arising out of a genetic condition known as 'Crie de Chat'. Despite the severity of his disability I have often described him as one of the least handicapped people that I have ever met.

Dylan's childhood was spent in a scattered hamlet in a rural coastal region in North Anglesey. Apart from time at home with his parents, much of his time was spent with his siblings and their friends. They played games and wandered across hedgerows and through fields with Dylan in tow. The children pursued their own interests but also, as a matter of course, accepted responsibility for Dylan and involved him, within his abilities, in their games and preoccupations.

In this context, Dylan was accepted as a person in his own right with both an acceptance and a disregard for his disabilities. While this description underlines the nature of his relationship with his peers, it also demonstrates the ability and trust of his mother in avoiding an overprotective approach and taking a well-assessed and robust attitude to risk taking.

Until he was about ten years old, he had no formal language, but his mother learnt about Makaton signing and set about teaching it to him. Dylan discovered that he could take a part in conversations and became even more socially involved.

When I first met Dylan, some six years ago, I was most impressed by his character. Despite limitations on his physical abilities, despite no speech, he appeared to have a very well-developed sense of himself. He was curious, often inconveniently demanding and, despite his inability to speak, he was, in relative terms, an excellent communicator. In the vernacular, he was a 'go-er'. If you were unable to understand his message, he would persist. He was a social person and a great mimic, and could give an excellent rendition of some of his schoolmates capturing their idiosyncrasies and character to a 't'.

During the time that I have known him his use of sign language has developed. Though much of his signing vocabulary was taught by his mother and others, he began to invent his own signs, with considerable ingenuity. Examples of such signs are pointing to the sky to denote 'The Boss', i.e. the manager of the daycare service he attended. Another example of his idiosyncratic signs was bending his arm upwards at the elbow and reaching his hand forward in a grabbing motion. This sign was an imitation of a JCB digger and signified the member of staff who drove the JCB.

Feelings he would express by grimaces, mock tears, etc.

I gained the strong impression that Dylan had much more to share than his disabilities allowed. Despite his limitations he endeavoured to converse and, depending on the motivation of his recipient, he usually succeeded to a good degree. He also seemed to understand what language was about. Though his signing vocabulary was very limited, he used it flexibly. In this sense his style of sign language use is quite different from the rather rigid use of signs that many people with a severe learning disability demonstrate. Dylan's 'normality' and 'conversationality' was not the product of formally planned and implemented programmes. Dylan's formative life experiences were natural. The important people involved in Dylan's life might look back and say that they might have done such and such a bit better. In terms of care giving there is no such thing as perfect care giving. If there were it would probably be quite unhealthy.

Child rearing is an impossible job. It is complex, intuitive and no parent will get it right. Donald Winnicott used the term 'good enough Mother' (Winnicott 1991). This term included not only the idea of the impossibility of the task but also the undesirability of doing a perfect job!

So, for the most part, Dylan became a member of society by learning naturally. His experience of the world was the result of fairly intuitive decisions, actions and accidents. The one thing that was not spontaneous was the adoption of Makaton. This was special needs type technology and it met a need. It allowed Dylan to become a much more competent conversationalist. Here again though there was an issue of style. Formal Makaton is a rigid stage-based system where the student is required to follow the systematic signing curriculum. Dylan's experience was different. He was given signs as and when he needed them for conversations. The signs were a means and not an end in themselves.

How do we help the 'unheard' to be heard

It is rather dangerous to make sweeping generalisations but my experience is that often language is taught or trained as a method of communication. As such it can be, and often is, an instrument of control. In the overconfident spirit of sweeping generalisation let me state a law!

'Where there is no conversation there is a struggle for control.'

As a corollary to this we might make the following statement:

'Where there is a struggle for control there is exotic communication.'

Further corollaries are:

'Where there is exotic communication there is pressure on service managers to spend money' and 'Conversations save money'.

Lest anyone thinks that psychologists are prone to megalomania in pronouncing laws, let me say that these aren't real laws. These are statements that should be lovingly copied using your best calligraphy pens, framed, and placed above your beds as objects of contemplation!

If we take Dylan's story as a demonstration of what is possible, perhaps as a sort of bench mark of Winnicott's 'good enough' we can begin to recognise some 'not good enough' deviations. The following come to mind, though more are possible:

1. not understanding the experience of the individual;
2. not understanding the nature of conversation;
3. denying the disability.

1. The experience of the individual

It seems likely that the experience of the world that the person with autism has is so different from ours that there may be little contact between our personal realities. In our attempts to communicate we can become troublesome and problematic for the person with autism. This does not necessarily mean that the person with autism does not need and want love and affection, they may be desperate for it. It may be that our attempts to provide this are inept and end up being aversive. I owe this insight to a colleague, Meena O'Neill, and to several clients including Daniel.

Daniel was autistic, had no speech, and no apparent interest in social interaction. His favoured activities were scooping gravel or small objects in his hand and watching intently as he poured them through his fingers onto the ground. I established contact with him by engaging him in the same game, by imitating his game. He became interested and animated in this style of interaction. Contact with him felt warm. He showed me that he liked the back of his neck massaged. A carer, with good contact with Daniel, told me that Daniel could be calmed down by this if he was stressed. One day Daniel was ill. He had diarrhoea and was in distress. He was crying. He reached for my hand and put it behind my neck asking for a massage. I complied and he immediately responded by digging his nails into my arm and pushing me away. As soon as he had pushed me away he pulled me back asking for a massage. Again he dug his nails in. This sequence persisted for a while. I found it distressing. He was obviously asking for comfort and I couldn't give it to him. I was making things worse and exacerbating his distress. I eventually found a blanket, wrapped him in it then retreated to a distance. Being held by the blanket seemed to calm him down. On subsequent occasions, when distressed he would seek out a blanket and swaddle himself.

I couldn't begin to understand Daniel's experiences. I was applying my own intuitions about his experience and needs and this was causing him distress. It was also causing me some distress, a bit like a mother trying to placate an inconsolable child. It was only when I stood back and refocused that I had any chance of resolving the situation.

2. The nature of the conversation and the danger of experts

If the person with learning disability is accepted as a person, along with his disabilities, then the danger of underestimating the person's capacity to communicate is minimised. Dylan's discovery of signing was in a sense accidental. His mother searched for answers to meet his needs. Had his mother lived in an urban setting then the opportunities to learn about signing systems would have been rich. Yet in an urban setting, the unfettered freedom of peer group play would have been more difficult. The degree of risk taking in allowing freedom to wander would have been irresponsible. Whatever the setting, the possibility of enabling the conversation is enhanced if needs are assessed, recognised, and the means to meet those needs are implemented. This requires 'expertise'. (I cannot resist sharing a definition of an expert which I will attribute to one A. Cashmore Thorley (personal communication). Expert: Ex; past it/ Spurt; a drip under pressure.)

Expertise is an essential yet dangerous commodity. People like clinical psychologists, speech therapists, special needs teachers, community nurses, physiotherapists, occupational therapists, psychiatrists, to name but a few, have had considerable training. They are asked to give advice so as to alleviate situations which are difficult, complex and distressing. They have much to contribute but they have no magic wands. Yet they are under enormous pressures to make things right.

The clinician who succumbs to this anxiety and pressure becomes the expert who tells people what to do. The carers, whether they are parents or staff are desperate to become 'perfect mothers'. They want the expert to be a perfect mother for them and to feed them with perfect programmes. They can become insatiable and demand more and more feeding. They can become very dependent on the expert. What the expert feeds them becomes the food that they feed the person who they care for. That person is subject to the task-oriented demands of the programme. He or she is not listened to and again is denied the opportunity for conversations.

The mother of a child with special needs will receive advice from a number of professionals. That advice often takes the form of a programme for the mother to follow. She may have at least as many different programmes as there are professionals visiting. All mothers feel guilty or inadequate at some time. Such feelings are a God-given feature of maternity. It is in the very nature of being 'good enough' and not being perfect. Disability, to my mind, acts as a magnifying glass on normal relationships. The mother of the child with a disability has to cope with the considerable and complex additional needs of her child. Unless there is an unusual degree of acceptance there is always the hope that their child might be made better. The professional entering the family gets sucked into these pressures and feels compelled to provide therapy. There is a script going on which is much more powerful than the players. The result is that everyone becomes stressed. When the child eventually goes to school, usually special school, mothers fall back into their armchairs in an exhausted state and say, 'Thank God. I can be a mother again!'.

It is only at this point that the mother has the luxury of allowing her offspring to be a conversationalist. Unfortunately, the effect of the input will have worked against conversations. The disabled child will have been denied the opportunities for conversation. On entering the special school, teaching staff will be under the pressures of goal-oriented professional approaches and will continue to engage in non-conversational approaches. The degree to which the individual teacher succumbs to such institutional pressure or follows their principles as a child-centred educator, depends on the culture of the school that they work in. This reflects the degree of sensitivity and support that their management provides. It reflects the degree of creativity with which the school translates SATS into meaningful conversational activities for the pupils. It reflects the sensitivity of the education authorities in recognising the centrality of conversational needs. There is nowadays, an unfortunate distinction between developmental needs and educational needs. On the one hand we have the playful, rather intuitive, yet informed nature of conversational approaches. On the other hand we have the more formal goal-oriented, more easily accountable, procedural approaches which are part of the current ethos.

Professional accountability is essential, but if we are to engage in rational exercise in providing feedback about our effectiveness then we need measuring instruments that are congruent with our aims of meeting the child's complex needs. Simple, unidimensional, numerical models only serve to distort reality and create a chasm between the professional care giver and their managers. Meanwhile, the child's real needs will not be addressed.

So how do we stop being experts and start being really useful?

Earlier I mentioned the carers who demand the expert to feed them with programmes. There may be some considerable expertise but there is no such thing as an expert in this field. The best that one might hope for is an experienced and sensitive advisor who has expertise. What does such a person do when confronted with demands for programmes? The answer is to engage in conversation with the carers. This might start initially by the advisor saying that the purpose of the first few visits is to get to know the client and the carers. This might entail some assessment but the emphasis is on 'getting to know you'. Part of this would entail the carers talking about themselves, their situation, their feelings about the client. Part of the process would be to engage in conversations with the client. This might entail getting down on the floor with a child or adult with profound disabilities and joining in with whatever preoccupations they might have. This conversation can become part of the conversation with the carers. The purpose is to help the carers to value and understand what the other person is doing. It may involve bringing in some expertise in the form of explanations, reasons for things happening. All being well, the carers may begin to involve themselves in conversations with the person. It often happens that the carers are already engaged quite naturally in conversations with the person. This is valued by the carers but they assume that others don't value such engagements. There is a sense that these conversations are private and intimate. The advisor needs to be sensitive to this but at the same time develop a relationship with the carers such that it becomes quite natural for him or her to be included in this intimacy. Where the carers are professional staff then there may be a feeling that such conversations are disapproved of. The sight of the advisor engaging in similar conversations serves to legitimise and value the staff's conversations.

Where there is need for more formal assessments or procedures then such tools can be brought in as part of the conversation with the carers. They remain partners in the enterprise and the tools have less danger of getting in the way of everyone's conversations.

3. Denying the disability

It sometimes happens that carers assume that the person with a learning disability is able to understand much more than they do. This is most likely to happen when that person is relatively able and has good social skills. It can happen, paradoxically, when parents are really tuned in and have really enabled their offspring to attain their potential. Often they will have attended mainstream schools and in the special needs class they have been quiet and compliant. They are quiet and compliant because they don't want anyone to get too close and catch them out. So all seems well until they come under obvious pressure. This can take different forms which might include being bullied, coping with the transfer to a college of further education, or being placed on work placements.

What transpires is that the person has been playing the part of a much more able person. They use language as if they understand, but if we tune in and listen carefully we might discover that this is an act. Behind this persona of a quiet and coping person the real person is chronically anxious and frightened of being caught out. Sometimes the anxiety can become so intense that the person cannot cope anymore. The facade breaks down and we are faced with a very distressed and disturbed person. The disturbance might be so extreme that we are tempted to use labels such as schizophrenia and multiple personalities. It is very difficult to help a person with this degree of disturbance, but they do need to withdraw and to be helped to negotiate a new and less stressful relationship with their world.

A person in this situation might be helped by discovering someone who can have a conversation with them. This is best sooner rather than later. Often when we talk to each other it is as if we are swimming in a sea of words, where we catch some meanings. If we are lucky we can ask the other, check out, ask for repetitions, so as to help us catch more of the meanings. Even then we can be helped by non-verbal methods. In a seminar, putting ideas and images on a flip chart can help us to anchor onto the image of what is being discussed. The same can work for someone who seems verbally able but where there are limitations on their apparent ability.

One of the areas that is often difficult to talk about is feeling. Often the person has learnt that it is only acceptable to be happy. They have been taught that to be angry or sad or whatever is not acceptable. They then have an understanding of happy. They will often maintain that they are 'happy' when they are not. The real feelings that they experience are confused and unlabelled. If there is a label then it is something like 'bad'. The sense of this 'bad' is 'I am bad for not being nice and happy'. Conversations which recognise and accept 'bad' feelings can be a new and unique experience which will help the person to accept themselves. These conversations are often helped by pictures, however crudely drawn, which help to provide images onto which these feelings can be anchored. Diagrams showing the most important people in a client's life can help to locate and explore feelings about these others, including oneself. At the core of this process is helping the person to accept themselves as being unique and valued.

This may involve talking about what Dr Joan Bicknell termed, 'The Three Taboos'. People have difficulty in talking to people with a disability about sex, death, and the disability itself. Accepting and celebrating each other's uniqueness involves accepting each other's needs as part of the whole person. A person who plays at being someone more able than themselves and who suffers an anxious dread of being 'caught out' is having their uniqueness denied. This leads us to another law.

'Where there is denial of the other's uniqueness, there is no conversation'.

The unloved and their scripts

The people that fall into this category are some of the most exotic communicators that carers and clinicians have to cope with. I have already begun to talk about people with bad feelings. When these feelings dominate every aspect of a person's life then it is those staff who tune into the person's stories who are likely to suffer. These staff are more likely to understand and accept the exotic and are in the best position to engage in conversation. Yet they are the ones who are most likely to receive the full and desperate fury of the person that they care for.

Jonathan was a young person, about 13 years old when I first knew him. He had spina bifida and because of this was incontinent and confined to a wheel chair. He also had epilepsy. Despite a high level of abilities he lived in a large hospital for people with a learning disability. He could read and write and was fairly numerate. His behaviour however, left much to be desired. He would hurl missiles at staff. His missiles included the contents of his incontinence pad, and his wheel chair. Knowing that a wheelchair might come flying across the room accompanied by a stream of invectives does little to encourage the prospect of a conversation. Most staff were wary and, at times, appropriately frightened of Jonathan. He was not a popular person.

Let's try and look at Jonathan growing up. As a three year old he would not have been walking, speech may have been slow in developing. His parents would be chronically anxious about his well-being. In those days child development teams did not exist, and so it is unlikely that his mum and dad had much formal and regular support. It seems likely that he would have seemed quite manipulative. He is likely to have been quite frustrated and prone to temper tantrums. His incontinence would also have added to the problem. By the time he was five his education would have been a problem. In those days provision was made in a range of special schools each with its own specialities. So where might Jonathan be placed? He was tried in several different settings. Each failed to meet his needs until eventually he was placed in, what was then termed, a subnormality hospital. His experience was that no one wanted him. He was dirty and had to wear nappies and everybody said that he was bad. He told me that he was put in the hospital because he was bad. It seemed that he believed everyone. Even in his own eyes he was dirty and bad.

People like Jonathan almost invariably find some people that become their allies. In Jonathan's case there was a core of about four of us. For some strange reason we liked him, despite his behaviour. This seemed to present problems for him. We became the focus of his attacks which were pretty physical. We coped as best as we could with this but somehow we still liked him. Sure, we were flesh and blood, and there were times when we were angry, but somehow we managed to contain our anger, and we stuck to him.

Our attitude presented a problem for Jonathan, possibly two problems. If he was so dirty and so bad, why did we like him? It just didn't make any sense. (Aside: Many of the unloved seem to deliberately spoil good things. They will break possessions which they value, they will spoil events, outings, etc. which they seem to be enjoying. To their carers this seems perverse and incomprehensible. Sometimes this may happen to someone who is obviously loved, without any history of rejection. It seems that such a person does not like themselves because of their disabilities. It is when they are reminded of their difficulties that spoiling behaviour becomes manifest.)

If Jonathan let us become close to him we might then just get rid of him and that would hurt. From his point of view, any relationship he had formed had been terminated when he was moved on. The safest bet was to keep us at bay. Our persistence possibly made things worse for him. Yet we persisted. Our approach was, 'We don't like the things that you do and we will respond appropriately, but that doesn't mean that we don't like you. We will stick with you because we like you.'

In effect we were splitting his behaviour from him as a person and helping him to build a new image of himself. Over a period of several years he changed. His exotic communications became less physical and more verbal. Instead of faeces we had exotic insults thrown at us, but gradually even those became less frequent. The last time I saw him he was in an adult education class writing about the plight of children in Somalia with a great deal of care and compassion.

Jonathan behaved as if he had a script which he had to follow. His script ran something like 'I'm a shit and nobody likes me. I don't want anybody to like me 'cos I'll be moved on anyway'. His experience was that his script was true because other people acted in accordance with his script, that is until he met a few who refused to follow his script. Jonathan's script was relatively straightforward. Trish's script was something else.

Trish was born angry. From day one she fought and screamed. Even feeding her was a battle. Her parents struggled and suffered with her. She eventually went to a local special school. She had some moderate learning disability and also some slight physical disability. There are memories of her spinning on her bottom in the classroom, lashing out with her leg brace at anyone who came close to her. In her mid teens her parents could cope no more and she was placed in a local hostel. Here the regime was tough but fair with very clear boundaries. There were very clear outcomes depending on whether her behaviour was 'good' or 'bad'. Within this regime she calmed down and began to develop good relationships with staff and with other people in the community. Eventually she was moved to a staffed community house, where she was a tenant with one other person. The approach in this setting was based on an interpretation of Wolfensburger's principles of normalisation. Trish's life was subject to her own choices so suddenly there were no boundaries. In one sense her situation was not dissimilar to a mythical first year undergraduate enjoying the excesses of life. She could not cope with this. She became increasingly difficult and disturbed and angry again. The project was obviously not viable and serious consideration was given to placing her 'out of county'. The local community nurse argued and wheeled and dealed with both Health and Social Services for a 'last chance' for Trish. His arguments were listened to and eventually accepted. So the 'last chance' project was set up.

The core of this project was the choice of staff that were to work with Trish – they were hand picked. They were warm and giving people with good intuitions and attitudes. They were all experienced in working with a number of clients who had quite difficult needs. They had almost all known Trish for many years and had worked with her. They were realistic about how difficult she could be and yet they all had a good relationship with her. They wanted to work with her. They were one of the best staff groups that I've worked with. Paul, the community nurse who had set the project up, was the project manager and I was his tame psychologist side-kick. We worked hard in providing the staff with further training. With the staff we worked out a very detailed care plan which provided Trish with a rich and varied lifestyle and the opportunity to develop her skills and capacity. We set up a very thorough staff support system which involved weekly staff meetings, regular and almost daily support visits, and an emergency on-call system for advice and support. Trish herself wanted the project to work. How could such a set-up fail?

A house was rented for the project and Trish moved in. Things went well for several months. When I say, went well, I do not mean it was easy. There were plenty of exotic incidents, struggles in maintaining boundaries which Trish would challenge with a vengeance. But after each such episode the good relationship between Trish and the staff team was reconfirmed.

In retrospect there was a specific day when there was a qualitative change in the project, when Trish no longer wanted the bloody thing to succeed. Looking back, she was tired and fed up with the lifestyle that we were providing. Looking back, it was too claustrophobic for her. (I have since become wary of single person projects, but that is the wisdom of hindsight.) Without the luxury of hindsight we carried on. Her attacks on staff became increasingly dangerous. Members of the community were in some risk of receiving her anger. The staff use of the emergency call system became increasingly frequent. Suddenly one day I had an insight. The relationship between Trish and staff had become exactly the same as the relationship between Trish and her Mum. They were desperately still trying to help her but this help had degenerated into a relentless nag. The staff team were exhausted and burnt out, just like mum.

Inevitably the project closed and Trish was placed in a special hospital, with the capacity to contain her anger. The staff moved on. They recovered and all continued to work with very difficult clients with warmth and humour.

Several years later I was giving a talk to a group of terrifyingly bright post-graduate psychologists. My talk was about models of service provision and included a description of the last chance project. I am a seasoned lecturer and workshopper. I feel that I consistently gain good rapport with my audience and come over as a warm and caring guy, but somehow this lot didn't like me. There was a wine and buffet session afterwards and I overheard one student say '. . . he didn't talk about the transference! (Transference is a term used in psychoanalysis to describe how the therapist experiences and recognises the client's feelings). It suddenly dawned on me that in the same way that the staff had become Trish's mother, Paul and I had become her father, defending and protecting the mother, the staff team, from her angry child. My audience of bright psychologists were receiving the vibes of this stern and angry father! Trish's script was still in operation.

Such scripts are invidious and powerful, especially when the emotional temperature of the client–carer relationship is high. For the sake of completeness, I will briefly mention another quite common script. It sometimes happens that a staff group may be split into two schools of thought about what is the right approach for a client. Such splits can be very divisive and feelings can run very strong. The client may be a piggy in the middle, or may well be manipulative and seem to enjoy the schism. Any such enjoyment is only apparent. As a psychologist I find working with such a split group very difficult. You might decide what the party line is and impose a three-line whip and expect people to fall into line. Such an approach tends to be subtly undermined.

Another approach is to take sides. The favoured side might feel self righteous. The psychologist, a powerful figure, is on their side. But then the losers are likely to be saboteurs, either deliberately or unconsciously.

Solutions work when staff own and believe in them. Although it can take a brave heart to take it on there is a lot to be said for setting up negotiation. Negotiation is initially about communication and, as I said earlier, communication is about power. There is a lot of power in knowing that you are right and the other is wrong. It is very difficult to move from a position of extreme self righteousness towards having a conversation with the other. Knowing that you are right is easier to live with than admitting that, though you are desperate to make somebody behave better, you haven't a clue. It's easier to blame things on those that don't agree with you. When this sort of thinking is going on, it's likely that old arguments between the client's mum and dad are still going on. The script is bigger than you. Such scripts make negotiation very difficult. The psychologist as arbitrator can make considerable headway by helping people to recognise and understand the nature of the script.

Back to the vunder of Venn

The careful reader will recall my vennphilia. So far I have described each circle in turn. The beauty of Venn diagrams is that they overlap so we can have those in pain and unheard, those unheard and unloved, those unloved and in pain. It will be apparent that in my discussion so far I have already indicated some of these combinations, but let me now introduce Phil. He was, in pain, unheard and unloved.

Phil was a child resident in a large institution. He was quite a character and gained the affection of most of the staff. He was stone deaf and quite mute. In relative terms he was quite an able boy. He was socially very astute. He could spot a behaviour modification programme a mile away. It seemed he could work out the rules and then take great joy in doing a slalom around them. Despite many years of being taught sign language he was unable to communicate with it. Given his level of ability, his sociability and his obvious need to communicate, this was surprising. Phil was a most likeable rogue, yet he could be impossible. There were times that his communicative inabilities made him frustrated and his exotic communications could be quite fierce. But these episodes were very short lived. Phil grew up into adolescence and probably as a result of this, his behaviour began to deteriorate.

Phil's mother was very fond of him but his condition was a source of great pain to her. During his teens she began to visit him more frequently. Phil and his Mum enjoyed the contact and so she began at weekends to take him home for the day. These outings went well so Phil now stayed for the entire weekend. The weekend stays proved successful, so Phil's mum discharged him so that he could stay permanently at home. After a few weeks the situation deteriorated and Phil was brought back. There would be no contact with his mother for several months. Then she would begin again to visit him in the hospital. These turned into days at home, then weekends at home, then discharge. This cycle happened several times. Phil became increasingly disturbed. He began to tear his clothes. He had two sets of clothes. One set was provided by the hospital. The other set was provided by his mother. He would go through periods when his hospital clothes were being destroyed. At other times it was clothing that his mother had brought which were destroyed. This seemed very much to reflect his ambivalence and confusion. Phil also began to destroy his relationships. The charge nurse on the ward had a very good relationship with Phil but he suddenly became the butt of Phil's anger. Phil seemed to work relentlessly and systematically on destroying that relationship. His friend the charge nurse became increasingly stressed and began to dread coming to work. He even began to be haunted by Phil in his dreams. It was eventually decided that he should not work directly with Phil. Phil now turned his attention to another member of staff with whom he was friendly. He now became the butt of Phil's attacks. It was his turn to be stressed. This process continued until the whole staff group were demoralised and frightened. At this point Phil was transferred to the medium security ward at the hospital.

During this period it became apparent that there were times that Phil's anger had a different quality. Staff described his eyes looking very different, almost as if he were possessed. They said that it felt that it was a completely different person.

It seems possible that what the staff were describing were episodes of temporal lobe epilepsy. Temporal lobe epilepsy manifests itself in strange changes of mood and behaviour. The temporal lobes are the part of the brain which include the centres for speech and language. It is highly likely that Phil suffered from brain damage in these particular areas. His inability to use speech or sign language was significant. Being stone deaf is extremely rare and is likely to be a result of damage to the part of the brain that receives the product of much processing between ear and cortex, rather than a difficulty in the sensory apparatus. We are all potentially epileptic. It depends on what may trigger an epileptic episode. Potential triggers include high temperatures, flashing lights, high stress levels, etc. It may be that the high stress levels that Phil was experiencing were triggers to these apparent episodes. All this is conjectural but if my formulation is right then his story becomes even more poignant.

If, as a youngster, his difficulty in processing speech had been recognised then a system, probably visual, could have been implemented to help him. His life would have been quite different and happier. His sociability and interest in people suggest that his earlier relationship with his mother was very good. Phil seems to have so wanted to communicate that his frustrations must have been considerable. His mother must have been so desperate in wanting to meet his needs, such that over the years her desperation led to her apparent irrationality which then hurt Phil so much. Phil's staff became caught in the script. The charge nurse's stress and pain were a reflection of the mother's pain. Though in one sense Phil became one of the unloved, in another sense he remained loved by everyone who had formed a relationship with him even though that love caused pain.

The pained, unheard and unloved carers

The carers of a person with exotic communication may have visitors, outsiders coming in and showing an interest in their situation. When the outsider, be it psychologist, community nurse, speech therapist, occupational therapist, physiotherapist, paediatrician, psychiatrist, music therapist, drama therapist, social worker, plumber or whatever comes in, they are confronted by a drama of prewritten scripts. Such a melee is pretty frightening. As I suggested earlier it is understandable if the outsider hides behind their expertise and comes in with their own agendas. In this situation the carers feel just as lonely as those who are neglected. They don't feel that their needs are being recognised. If they don't comply with the outsider's agenda they are labelled difficult parents or a 'difficult staff group'. Communication with them is exotic and they may be perceived as being more difficult than the client. When this happens the carers can be neglected. No-one knows what to do so no-one comes. The carers are alone and lonely in their struggle to meet the needs of their exotic communicator.

The carers have become those in pain, unheard and unloved.

Working with people who communicate exotically can cause great stress and pain to carers whether they are parents or professional carers. This is particularly and poignantly so when they still admit to caring. It is because they care that they are prone to be hurt. It can happen that carers cannot bear the pain any more. They become defended against the pain. The person in their care ceases to be seen as a person and becomes an object or an alien. At an extreme, such objects can become subjected to inhumane practices and there is a sickness in the whole situation. This is one of the consequences of what is sometimes termed 'staff burn-out'.

Outmoded institutions such as ATCs and hospitals can be thought of as the palaeolithic remains of ancient models dreamt up by now forgotten social administrators. Staff working in these settings may be caught in ancient institutional scripts which we call the culture of the institution. One big script in the culture is that of 'primaeval burn out', where practices evolved which served to defend burnt-out staff. Such practices became normal and unremarkable but such practices dehumanise both staff and client.

I began this chapter by talking about Edward. You may recall that some staff perceived him as being psychotic. The effect of this label was to make him into an alien, a dangerous object. And he was treated as such. Yet in the same institution there were groups of staff who established and maintained a conversational relationship. Nowadays there are many institutions where the majority of staff are conscious of the nature of the institution and work hard to make the lives of their clients as rich and valued as possible. Such staff are rewarding and good colleagues to work with. But what about 'difficult staff'?

How to love 'difficult staff'!

Nowadays it is commonplace to talk about 'positive approaches to people with challenging behaviour', so why not adopt this approach to difficult staff and look for ways to engage at a conversational level? The starting point for this process is to recognise and appreciate their experiences and their settings. Let them know that you are listening and understand their problems and stresses. Don't patronise. Don't just sit there making sympathetic noises. Listen, not just to their stories, but to their feelings. They'll soon know whether you're really listening or not. If they know you're listening then you've got a conversation, you've got their trust. Then, through staff support and training you can help them to become conscious of the scripts of their own institution as well as the scripts of the individuals in their care. Be honest. Make your own agendas public, transparent and open to discussion. Finally, get out your calligraphy set. Lovingly and carefully write out the words of an old North American Indian proverb and put it above your bed for contemplation. The proverb . . .?

Well . . . *Don't criticise your neighbour 'till you've walked in his moccasins!*

References

Caldwell, P. and Flynn, M. (1995) *Towards Understanding: Ways of Working with People with Severe Learning Disabilities and Extensive Support Needs.* London: Pavilion.

Caldwell, P. (1996) *Getting in Touch: Ways of Working with People with Severe Learning Disabilities and Extensive Support Needs.* Brighton: Pavilion Publishing/Joseph Rowntree Foundation.

Ephraim, G. W. (1986) 'A brief introduction to augmented mothering', *Playtrac Pamphlet, Harperbury Hospital, Radlett/Herts.*

Kroese, S., Dagnan, G., Loumis, K. (eds) (1997) *Cognitive Behaviour Therapy for People with Learning Disability.* London: Routledge.

McGee, J. J., Menolascino, M. D., Hobbs, D. C., Menousek, P. E. (1987) *Gentle Teaching. A Non-Aversive Approach to Helping Persons with Mental Retardation.* New York: Human Sciences Press.

Nind, M. and Hewett, D. (1994) *Access to Communication: Developing the Basis of Communication with People with Severe Learning Difficulties through Intensive Interaction* London: David Fulton Publishing.

Oswin, M. (1981) *Bereavement of Mentally Handicapped People.* London: King's Fund.

Oswin, M. (1984) *They Keep Going Away.* London: King's Fund.

Rogers, C. R. (1990) *On Becoming a Person.* London: Constable.

Sinason, V. (1992) *Mental Handicap and the Human Condition, New Approaches from the Tavistock.* London: Free Association Books.

Sperber, D. and Wilson, D. (1986) *Relevance: Communication and Cognition.* Oxford: Blackwell.

Winnicott, D. M. (1991) *The Child, The Family, and The Outside World.* Harmondsworth: Penguin.

Author index

Subject index